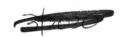

D1300573

BETTER
STRETCHING

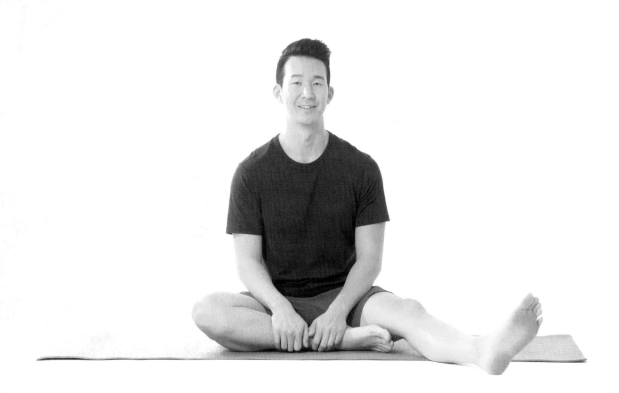

BETTER
STRETCHING

9 Minutes a Day

to Greater Flexibility, Less Pain,
and Enhanced Performance,
the JoeTherapy Way

Joe Yoon

ST. MARTIN'S
ESSENTIALS
NEW YORK

First published in the United States by St. Martin's Essentials, an imprint of St. Martin's Publishing Group

BETTER STRETCHING. Copyright © 2020 by Joe Yoon. All rights reserved. Printed in the United States of America. For information, address St. Martin's Publishing Group, 120 Broadway, New York, NY 10271.

www.stmartins.com

Designed by Steven Seighman

The Library of Congress Cataloging-in-Publication Data is available upon request.

ISBN 978-1-250-24821-3 (hardcover)
ISBN 978-1-250-24822-0 (ebook)

Our books may be purchased in bulk for promotional, educational, or business use. Please contact your local bookseller or the Macmillan Corporate and Premium Sales Department at 1-800-221-7945, extension 5442, or by email at MacmillanSpecialMarkets@macmillan.com.

First Edition: March 2020

10 9 8 7 6 5 4 3 2 1

This book is dedicated to everyone who has supported me throughout my journey, from my closest friends and family to those who know me through my work. The biggest thank-you goes to my mom. I couldn't have done any of this without your support. Love you, Mom!

CONTENTS

BETTER

STRETCHING

— INTRODUCTION

"I am tight." I hear those three little words on a regular basis. And I hear them from people whose day-to-day activities have little in common. Athletes are tight. Desk workers are tight. Stay-at-home parents are tight. Food servers are tight. Performers are tight. Pain and discomfort due to inflexibility is the great equalizer. Almost everybody experiences it in some form. If you picked up this book, chances are you feel tight, too.

Stretching can help. With regular stretching, muscles have greater give. They elongate more easily when you need them to, which not only allows you to accomplish any task with more grace and efficiency—whether that task is to reach up and grab a jar off a shelf or to extend your leg over a finish line—but to do so with a lower risk of injury. With well-stretched muscles, you are less likely to suffer from the body imbalances that lead to back, knee, hip, and shoulder pain. And when you take the time to stretch, you can get rid of the tightness that comes from the demands of our modern-day world: sitting (tough on the back and lower body), hunching over a computer (oh, your aching shoulders!), and neck bent over a smartphone (the source of endless cricks).

So how much time? Nine minutes. Nine! That's it. If you have ever contemplated starting a stretching routine but dismissed the idea because you didn't have the time, that excuse is now null and void. Everyone has nine minutes.

The promise of this book is simple: You can achieve life-changing results for your body—greater mobility, improved functionality, better performance, less pain, and pain prevention—in as little as nine minutes a day. No ninety-minute yoga workouts, no belabored regimens that will have you flashing back to your mean high school gym teacher. Just a few targeted, feel-good moves and you're good to go.

I am a certified personal trainer and licensed massage therapist, and I have worked with many well-known athletes, including NFL Super Bowl champions, NFL Pro Bowlers, and multiple Olympic gold and world champions. I have also traveled the world with sprinter and Olympic gold medalist Justin Gatlin, serving as his stretching trainer and massage therapist. This work has given me a lot of insight into the needs of people who place high demands on their bodies. But what influenced me most as I developed the stretching plans for this book was the feedback I've received from the one-million-plus mostly everyday people who follow my Instagram account, JoeTherapy.

When I started posting on Instagram, there were already plenty of stretching videos available on the app. I made the decision to keep my videos a lot simpler than the ones already online because I firmly believe that simple does the trick. For everybody. Someone who sits in front of a computer all day will benefit from the same uncomplicated moves as an Olympic gold medalist. What's more, while it's nice to know the name of the muscle you're stretching, you don't need to understand the finer points of an anatomy textbook to get great results from a stretching routine.

This straightforward approach has clearly resonated with people, which is why I have followed the same game plan in crafting this book. It goes much further than my Instagram posts—besides presenting individual exercises, I have created routines for specific purposes as well as three thirty-day jump-start plans—but the stretches are easy and fast; there's no deep dive into anatomical science; and the exercises are as effective for desk workers as they are for weekend warriors and professional athletes.

This book also aims to familiarize you with all the things that not only increase flexibility but help you sustain it. One of those things is consistency. While simple stretches can do wonders for aching shoulders, relax a rigid back, and loosen up knotty calves, their effects can be fleeting if you don't do them regularly. But knowing that it will take only nine minutes out of your day, that's not a particularly tall order. By keeping the routines short, I hope to inspire you to do them on a daily basis. The more consistent you are, the better they work.

There are two other aspects of sustaining flexibility that I will also introduce you to in the upcoming pages. One of them is mobility. It's not just our muscles that determine how easily we can move; the joints play a critical role as well. Maybe you are flexible enough to touch your toes, but that doesn't mean you can lengthen your stride when you need to scramble to catch a toddler or run for a bus about to close its doors. It doesn't mean that you'll be able to glide side to side across a tennis court to pick up a shot to your backhand. Mobility exercises—the kind you'll find included in this book—are a type of stretching that promotes flexibility by increasing the joints' range of motion. Where typical stretches are passive, mobility exercises are active. You'll learn more about them in chapter 1.

The other important aspect of sustaining flexibility is strengthening. Most people don't know that a tight muscle could be a weak muscle. Lacking strength, muscles tend to tense up to protect themselves and the anatomical structures they surround. This doesn't mean you have to adopt a rigorous strength-training regimen (which isn't a bad thing—just not essential) to retain the gains you make by stretching, but adding in a spoonful of strengthening to your stretching routine can make a big difference in how loose and comfortable you feel in your body. I'll address this topic in more depth beginning on page 133, and in chapter 11, you'll find an assortment of simple but effective strengthening exercises to add to your stretching routine.

I've also included a chapter on how to use tools like foam rollers and self-massage balls. They can increase flexibility short term and have other related benefits, such as increasing circulation, which helps improve range of motion. Using these tools also feels really good, enough of a reason to try them if you haven't already. In chapter 12 I help you learn how to use them properly.

If you sit at a desk most of the day and find that every time you get up to walk down the hall you're hobbled by tightness, this book will help you loosen up. If you're a high-level athlete looking to improve the range of motion in your hips, this book has you covered. And if you're somewhere in between—unyielding calves are messing up your weekly pickup game of basketball, or after carrying your dog from the car to the veterinarian's office you're waking up with a stiff spine—there's a perfect stretch routine waiting for you here as well, no matter what shape you're in or body type you have.

PART 1

STRETCHES AND MOBILITY EXERCISES

— 1

WHAT YOU NEED TO KNOW ABOUT STRETCHING

The physiology behind stretching is fascinating—if you're a physical fitness geek like I am. But I'm willing to bet that most of you would prefer to skip the detailed anatomy lesson and just, so to speak, get on with the show: the stretching exercises themselves. Fortunately, you don't need to know much about what makes the muscles and joints work to get the most out of this book, so I'm not going to take you through a long and detailed explanation of cell biology. I do, however, want to introduce you to some basic facts about stretching and give you a few simple guidelines to follow. There are also many myths and misconceptions about stretching that could use some clearing up. I'll do that here as well as present some stretching-related concepts that you might not have heard about before.

There are certain questions that people ask me over and over again: Is it risky to stretch a cold muscle? What can I do to make the pain in my (insert aching body part here) go away? Should I stretch before I exercise or after? I'm not surprised that there's so much confusion surrounding these and other issues. There are many schools of thought out there, and a lot of nuance gets lost in trying to make stretching recommendations one-size-fits-all. If you've read widely about stretching or watched a variety of YouTube videos, you may feel as though you've heard conflicting advice.

On the following pages, I'll give you my take on what constitutes the best approach to stretching, including when, why, and how to do it. Ultimately, you will be the authority on what works for your body. But everyone needs to start somewhere, and these explanations and recommendations—when combined with the detailed exercises and routines later in the book—will give you all the information you need to develop the nine-minute-a-day program that best suits your goals and body type. I promise to keep it short and sweet.

Let's start at the beginning. People usually stretch because they feel "tight." But how do we get that way in the first place?

I define *tight* as when getting your body (or parts of your body) into a certain position or moving in a particular way is more difficult than usual. Say that you wake up first thing in the morning and typically stretch your arms overhead, no problem. But on one particular morning, that usual feel-good stretch actually feels kind of bad, and it's a bit of an effort to get your arms all the way overhead. There's a stiffness to your shoulder joints and arm muscles. Or maybe you go out for a run and your stride feels shortened and clunky; your hamstrings don't seem as willing to move as easily as the day before. That's tight. How uncomfortable or even painful that tightness feels can vary. Tightness is pretty much a subjective feeling. But I'd say that most of us are all too familiar with the sensation.

What causes tightness? One of the reasons muscles and joints stiffen up is because, in this modern society, most people simply don't move enough. We don't use our bodies to their utmost potential and in the ways that we're genetically programmed to use them. Our joints have a pretty good range of motion, and our muscles can elongate fairly far when we need them to, but if we don't take advantage of those two attributes, we lose them—not entirely, but enough to where our movements may be restricted and feel uncomfortable.

Tightness can also be caused by the body adapting to how you *do* use it. For instance, if you sit for hours at a time, your hip flexors—the muscles that lift your knees up—will be in a shortened position for a lengthy duration. And your body gets used to it. It thinks it's the muscles' normal position. The result is that your hip flexors stay somewhat shortened when you finally move out of the seated position, making it difficult to stand up straight and perhaps even causing your lower back to arch to compensate for the imbalance.

Another factor in declining muscle flexibility has to do with aging. As the body ages, the joints don't conduct fluid as well as they used to, and that affects (as lack of fluid would suggest) the fluidity of our movements. Many people as they grow older don't move as much and that can have a domino effect, contributing to bone loss, muscle loss, and lack of strength, all of which can make you feel tighter. That last element—lack of strength—in particular can contribute to reduced flexibility in people of any age. I'll address that further on in this chapter.

Stretching helps counter tightness by allowing muscles to lengthen, "resetting" your body. But consistency is important.

Muscles can contract, which means they can shorten, and they can stretch, which means they can elongate. As I have just noted, holding your body in one position for extended periods of time and/or not using it to its fullest causes shortening. Stretching is the obvious antidote, a way to return the muscles to a healthier and more comfortable state. When you stretch, the muscles don't "grow" longer, but they do extend closer to their full range. If you do this often enough, the body gets used to it, and the brain says, "It's safe to stay in this elongated position." This is why you should stretch.

But let me make an even stronger case for it. Stretching is another piece of the healthy-life pie. Especially as you age and your muscles lose some of their natural suppleness and resiliency, stretching can improve your life by allowing your body to a) simply move more, and b) move in ways that it doesn't usually have occasion to. Remember, use it or you will lose it! Something else to remember about stretching is that some stretching exercises, including many of those in this book, enhance your mobility.

It's great to be flexible enough to touch your toes or maybe if you're really flexible even do the splits. But the most important reason to gain flexibility is that it helps you move more easily in real life. It's not so much that you can do the neat trick of touching your toes but that you can easily pick up something you dropped on the floor, or bend down and hoist up your kid without throwing your back out. If you're naturally flexible, you can be more agile on a tennis or basketball court, throw a ball with less effort, be more likely to reach a hat stored high on a shelf (and without pulling a muscle). You will glide, not shuffle, down the hall to your boss's office, ascend stairs with greater lightness, and decrease your times and improve your moves in your sport of choice.

Besides giving you a flexibility and mobility upgrade, stretching has a definite pleasure factor. If you have ever stretched before, even in the most casual of ways like rolling your neck after watching a long movie or splaying your legs out straight after driving for a few hours, you know it feels good. Stretch on a regular basis and you can get more of that pleasurable feeling, decrease tension in your body, and reduce discomfort.

Note the words *regular basis*. The effects of stretching can be improved over time if you stretch every day or every other day (or at the very least every third day). If you're just stretching on an as-needed basis whenever a particular part of your body feels stiff, the effects will most likely be short term. You can't lift weights in January and expect the effects to last through July. Same thing here. You need to practice stretching on an ongoing and consistent basis if you want to see improvements—and want those improvements to last.

Doing some strengthening work will boost the effects of your stretching routine.

Strength is an often overlooked component of flexibility and mobility. Sometimes muscles become tight because they're weak. When a muscle lacks strength, your body will find a way to protect it. Think, for instance, about what happens when you're threatened in some way or find yourself falling. Your muscles tense up. It's the same thing when your body feels weak; your muscles stiffen to compensate for the lack of strength. That's the reason I have included a chapter on strengtheners in this book. Through some resistance training—not even full-on weight training, just some exercises that mostly use your own body weight—you can reinforce the gains you make through stretching and avoid weaknesses that lead to tight muscles.

Strengthening exercises are primarily designed to deliver on their name—they build strength. But most of them actually have a built-in stretching component, too. One part of a resistance exercise is called an *eccentric contraction*, and it involves actively lengthening the muscle. When you do a push-up, the effort you make to lower your body to the ground stretches your chest muscles. That's eccentric, muscle elongation. The part where you push yourself back up contracts the chest. That's called a *concentric contraction*. In a biceps curl, the concentric move is when you're lifting the weight toward your shoulder. The eccentric move is when you're lowering the weight back down. These and other strengthening moves don't replace stretches, but in the long run, they can help you avoid tightness and improve your flexibility.

There are several different stretching techniques. These are the three most common.

I don't think one way of stretching is better than any other. The stretching technique you should use depends on what your goals are. Is, for instance, your stretching routine part of your preworkout warm-up? Are you just aiming to alleviate tightness from sitting in a meeting too long? You can address these intentions with different ways of stretching.

Two of the three methods I describe below, static and dynamic stretching, are the primary ones used in this book. The third method, called contract-and-relax, builds on static stretching and can be used in place of it if it feels good to you. Here is how the three methods stack up.

STATIC STRETCHING. This is probably what you think of when you think of stretching. It involves passively holding a position without moving for anywhere from fifteen seconds to two minutes. Picture a typical standing hamstring stretch: You prop your leg up on a table, then bend your upper body over the raised leg and reach your arms toward (or, if possible, grab on to) your toes. A static hamstring stretch asks just that you stay there for a while in a fairly passive position, allowing the muscle to elongate to the point where you can feel tugging and a little discomfort (though it generally and strangely also feels pretty good), but it doesn't hurt.

DYNAMIC STRETCHING. This technique calls for actively moving the joints back and forth through a complete range of motion. The movements are controlled—not like ballistic stretching, which involves bouncing in and out of position—and fairly natural. One example is the T-Spine Windmill Stretch (Half-Kneeling) on page 91. In this stretch, you kneel with your arms out in front of you, then swing one arm upward in a half circle until it's behind you. As you go, your chest will rotate to the side. You then bring your arm back in front of you and repeat on the other side. In this stretch, you are not only lengthening your muscles, you are taking the shoulder joint through a range of motion, loosening it up so you ultimately move better.

CONTRACT-AND-RELAX STRETCHING. This technique works like this: You stretch a muscle just as you do in static stretching, holding it to the point where it starts to feel a little bit uncomfortable. Next, you contract that muscle (tighten it up) for a few (two to five) seconds, then release it. Repeat several times. Whenever you move into a static stretch, your muscle will eventually resist the stretch. You'll feel it when you reach that point, and that will determine how far into a stretch you go. But when you contract the muscle as you hold it, as you do in this technique, it tricks the muscle into letting up on the resistance and relaxing so when you release the contraction, you'll be able to move farther into the stretch. For instance, if you went back to that hamstring stretch I described earlier in the static stretching section and, instead of just passively hanging out over the leg for the whole time, alternatingly contracted and relaxed your hamstrings a few times, you'd stretch farther toward your toes than if you just held the stretch in a static position. Contract-and-relax stretching is a good way to get an intenser stretch.

When is the best time to stretch?

The best time to stretch is when you know you'll do it. Just fit it in. Some people like to do their stretch routine at 5:00 a.m.; others like to stretch at 9:00 p.m. It doesn't matter. If you are exercising, you may want to tack your stretching routine onto your workout (see below). Knock out two birds with one stone. Again, consistency is the most important aspect of stretching, so make that the deciding factor when you set your schedule.

Stretching can—and should—be combined with other types of exercise.

One of the most confusing issues surrounding stretching is how it figures into an overall exercise program. Maybe you've heard that it's important to stretch before you exercise but that it's not as important to stretch after you're done. Or maybe you've heard the opposite, that you should forget stretching before exercise—it may even inhibit your performance—but be sure to stretch after your workout.

Although research is being done on pre- and postexercise stretching, right now, there is not enough evidence to prove that one way is right and one way is wrong. Let me give you my opinion based on the experience I've had working with both athletes and everyday exercisers.

Yes, you should do *dynamic* stretches before you work out. Because it gets you moving in ways that are slightly more vigorous than static stretching, dynamic stretching warms up your core body temperature, which makes your muscles more elastic and preps them for the demands you'll soon be making on them. Even better if you do dynamic stretches that mimic the movements you'll be using in your workout. For instance, the T-Spine Windmill Stretch (Half-Kneeling) I mentioned earlier is perfect for swimmers because it gets the shoulder joints prepped and simulates the core rotation called for by many strokes.

Should you never static stretch before exercising? If you like to do some stretches where you hold a position, it's not the end of the world. Some of the better research has shown static stretching before exercise can decrease power somewhat, but is that something you really care about? And even if that gives you pause, consider that unless you plan to, say, put in a weight lifting session where you go the max, static stretching before you push off on your bike for a ride, or hit the track for a jog isn't going to make that big of a difference.

What others worry about is injury. I don't think you are likely to hurt yourself if you do a few static stretches before exercising as long as you always ease your way into a static stretch instead of going at it forcefully. Sink rather than dive into it. This goes for dynamic stretches as well. When I do them, I start by barely bending my knees or rotating my body. As my routine progresses, I start to push it a bit. Here, though, is the main rule of thumb: Listen to your body. If it's vigorously resisting movement, that's a sign that you need to back off. If you feel as though walking for a few minutes to get your body temperature up helps make stretching easier, go for it. We all have different levels of flexibility, and we don't all warm up at the same speed. A high school kid can walk into a gym, do a bench press at full weight right off the bat, and walk out happy and unscathed. I, on the other hand, need to warm up for ten to fifteen minutes, lift less weight than my maximum for a few reps, and work my way up to my full challenge. Your own plan of action will depend on who you are.

As for stretching *after* exercise, it's not a must but is perfectly fine. There has been some suggestion in the past that stretching after you work out helps decrease muscle soreness, and there's a chance that it does (though there's no hard evidence). In any case, stretching provides a nice way to cool down and relax after pushing yourself.

Stretches can help, but they are not a cure-all for pain.

If you feel tight in a particular area and you also feel pain in that area, it's logical to blame the pain on the tightness. Sometimes there may in fact be a cause-and-effect relationship between the two, but not always. The pain could be caused by something else entirely—maybe the area is inflamed, or lack of strength is the issue. The pain may even be contributing to your stiffness.

People often believe that if they just had the right stretch to take away the tightness, the pain would go away as well. I'm often asked to recommend stretches for a particular ache or pain, and there's a good chance that many of you, too, will find yourself thumbing through these pages looking for relief from some twinge or throbbing you're experiencing. So let me explain my approach to using stretching for pain relief.

Stretching is a great tool for keeping your body balanced and supple so you feel lighter and more limber and ultimately avoid injury and other painful conditions. If you are already in pain, stretching also has the potential to make you feel better, at least for a little while—as long as you do it gently and don't push yourself too far. But for the most part, stretching is not a cure-all for pain. The reasons we feel pain can be complex, so if you're hurting badly, or it's just not going away, you don't want to put a Band-Aid on it. Most sore muscles heal with time and nothing else, so try just giving an achy body part some rest. If it continues to hurt, you are in acute pain, or have swelling, make sure to have it checked out by a professional. Stretching might be part of the healing process, but you want to make sure you're getting to the bottom of the problem.

One place where stretching can also potentially help is with post workout muscle soreness. Some people feel tight after they've put in a particularly grueling workout. Tightness may indeed be the case, but what they perceive as tightness may also just be muscle soreness, another thing entirely. Still, stretching can be a remedy for both. Because it increases the circulation, and because it gets muscles used to moving again, stretching can help alleviate aches while also helping the body loosen up.

The same basic stretches work for just about everybody.

If a client who jogs tells me he occasionally has limited flexibility in his hips, I give him the same hip flexor stretch as I'd give a professional sprinter who is also tight in the hips. There may be some slight variation to accommodate different levels of flexibility, but the basic stretch is the same. Even if the goals are different—sprinters may want to lengthen their stride, joggers may just want to alleviate some tension that's causing discomfort—the exercises used to achieve them don't need to be. What this means is that you don't have to worry about whether the stretches in this book are too advanced or not advanced enough for your needs. With a few tweaks (and you'll find tips on how to make stretches easier or intenser throughout), they work for everybody.

When putting the stretches together, use the 4 + 1 formula and consider your goals.

In the upcoming chapters, you will be presented with more than a hundred stretches, mobility exercises, and strengtheners. Of course, you're not going to do all of them (that would take a lot longer than nine minutes!), so which ones do you choose? If you like things laid out for you or have a particular goal in mind, you will find seven nine-minute routines in chapter 12, each designed for a specific purpose. The jump-start routines in the appendix of this book also put the stretches together for you in a way that lets you make progress over a thirty-day period. If, however, you'd like to create a stretching routine on your own, here are a few recommendations for choosing exercises and stringing them together in an effective way.

1. *The formula.* To keep your routine to nine minutes, **choose four stretches or mobility exercises plus one strengthener** (foam-rolling exercises, which you'll read about in chapter 11, are extracurricular—if you add them in, your routine may go longer than nine minutes). I suggest that you do the same routine **every day for a week**, which will give you a chance to build on the gains you make. With consistency, you are going to get results. After a week, you may want to change it up so you don't get bored, but don't leave your old routine completely behind or you may lose the gains you made. You might, for instance, create a second routine that you alternate with the first one. If you find you have more than nine minutes to spare, simply add in more exercises, bearing in mind that strengthening can help you get more out of your stretches (in other words, when you add, add strengtheners, too).

2. *Whole-body stretching.* What would an ideal routine look like? It's tempting to just, say, focus on stretching your legs if you're a runner, or to choose only exercises that get the crick out of a neck victimized by too much computer time. But I urge you to spend the nine minutes a day you devote to stretching doing a variety of moves. Sure, hit any area that may be giving you trouble, but also try to extend

beyond that body part to give others the care they need, too. Try to think of your body as a whole. Everything is connected, so give everything its due.

How this ultimately comes together will vary. One approach that I like to use is to begin with stretches for the spine and hips, then add in ones for the extremities. On a given day, my own personal program might begin with something like the (1) T-Spine Cat/Cow Stretch (page 83), which loosens up the mid- and upper back. I then move on to a (2) stretch for the hips and glutes (such as Pigeon Pose, page 65), add in (3) a mobility exercise for the chest and shoulders (like the Dynamic Pec Stretch (Half-Kneeling), page 110), (4) a Wide-Legged Hamstring Stretch for the legs (page 41), and (+1) the Deadbug exercise (page 138) for core strengthening.

There's no one right way to do a stretch.

Every stretch I introduce you to in this book will have instructions on how to do it properly, with tips to make sure you get the most out of the move as well as avoid injury while doing it. So what do I mean that there's no right way to do a stretch?

Stretching allows for creativity. There is no reason that while you're doing a stretch for, say, your hamstrings, you can't also add a reach or a rotation or a side bend to make the move multifaceted. For example, to do the Triceps Stretch (Standing) (page 117), you sit cross-legged and use one hand to pull on the elbow of the other arm to get a stretch in the triceps (back of the upper arm). Now, what if while you are holding the stretch, you bend to the left? You'll also get a great stretch down the side of your body.

As you get to know the different ways to stretch, go off the reservation a bit. Try making modifications that allow you to maximize your time investment. Naturally, don't do anything that hurts—that's the ironclad rule—but be adventurous. It will pay off.

Nine minutes of stretching a day is enough for overall good health and fitness. If your goals are higher, do more.

How flexible do you need to be? That is a question only you can answer, and it depends on what you hope to accomplish. If you want to increase your reach in basketball or tennis, get more competitive at golf, get faster times in a triathlon, or be nimbler on the black diamond slopes, you may need to do more than nine minutes a day. But for the average person who just wants to feel and perform better (even if by "performing" you're just walking up several flights of stairs without difficulty), nine minutes is the perfect place to start. Yet feel free to *stretch* the time out as you get more proficient at the exercises. I think you'll enjoy having that feel-good time to yourself.

A few last things before you get started.

BREATHING. It's a good thing! Definitely remember to breathe while you are holding your stretches. In yoga, stretches are often coordinated with the breath. You don't have to worry about that so much when doing the exercises in this book, but you may find it helps ease your movements if you inhale before you move into a stretch, then exhale as you extend. As you're holding the stretch, breathe normally, perhaps going deeper into the stretch as you exhale. Whatever you do, don't hold your breath.

A "GOOD STRETCH." In the stretch instructions, I often use the phrase *until you feel a good stretch.* What I mean by that is you should feel a tug in the targeted muscle(s) that is maybe a little uncomfortable but doesn't hurt. It may even be pleasurable. In any case, you want to really *feel* the move. That's what lets you know it's working.

TARGET AREAS. While each exercise is devoted to a particular body part, each also has what you might call a *collateral advantage*—that is, almost every one of them also works other muscles as well. They don't work them as well as stretches where those secondary muscles are the main event, but they do give you some bonus bodywork.

REPETITIONS. Some of the dynamic stretches (exercises where you move rather than hold for a long period) call for repetitions or "reps." Most stretches, however, ask that you do only one repetition. Yep, that's it! You are welcome to do more than one rep as time and willingness allow, but take comfort in knowing that one does the job.

HOW OFTEN. To reiterate, since you need to stretch only for nine minutes, I suggest you do it every day. Yes, every day. It's only nine minutes! There's no reason not to. And I can guarantee you, it's going to feel good.

LOOKS AREN'T EVERYTHING. Every person's body is different. There are a range of body types and variations within those body types, so if you don't look exactly like I do when we're doing the same stretch or exercise, don't be concerned. It doesn't necessarily mean you're doing it wrong.

There is a host of factors that determine small differences in body position, including innate flexibility and the way an individual body is built. For instance, I'm six foot two and have long limbs, so when I do a squat, my upper body wants to tip forward. Someone who has shorter legs and different hip anatomy might be able to squat with a perfectly upright torso. Many people have a naturally rounded midback, while others have a super-straight midback. A rounded midback may make it a little tougher to fully rotate your shoulders and get your arms overhead during certain exercises. Use the photos as a general guideline when you do the exercises, but the best gauge is how you feel in a stretch. If it's working, you'll know it.

— 2

STRETCHES FOR THE LOWER LEGS

The major muscles of the legs, the quadriceps and the hamstrings, tend to get a lot of attention. And they should; they're the workhorses of the body, propelling us forward and backward. But the muscles in the lower legs also play an important role in mobility, helping us pivot and move side to side. For a healthy, flexible body, you need a healthy, flexible foundation, which is why the lower legs—which carry so much of our weight—are also worth paying considerable attention to.

I consider the "lower leg" to be the area beneath the knee, which includes the feet and toes—both of which tend to be overlooked when it comes to stretching. These smaller muscles also tend to get abused a bit. Besides carrying our weight, they get shoved into shoes, sometimes have to contend with the strain of wearing heels, and are subject to pounding on pavement and irregular surfaces. This leaves them vulnerable to injuries like ankle twists, calf and foot cramps, and Achilles strains. The lower legs, in other words, definitely warrant some TLC. You'll find the exercises you need to give it to them in the next few pages.

Feet and Toes

Stretching should start literally from the ground up, which means your feet and toes. I want to stress how important these body parts are in the grand scheme of things. Take the super-underrated big toe. The big toe helps control balance and can affect the way we walk, run, sprint, and perform many other movements. The rest of the foot is integral to how we move, too, but encased in hard and narrow shoes, sometimes all day, the foot and toes begin to stiffen and lose the ability to move in the way they should. If you can keep these little guys mobile, it can help the way your whole body moves overall, improve pain symptoms, and enhance your athleticism.

WHAT ARE YOU IMPROVING?
Mobility in the toes and feet.

ADDED BENEFIT
Reduces the aching that comes from a long day of standing or pounding the pavement.

FOOT STRETCH
(Kneeling)

I never used to think much about my feet. But then sharp pains and discomfort started to pop up here and there. That got my attention! Many people are bothered by plantar fasciitis and other foot problems but don't know how to ease the pain. I suggest starting here. This is a very simple stretch I use to give my feet a little love.

HOW TO DO IT: Kneel on the floor with your toes tucked under, heels up. Slowly shift your hips back so your butt rests on your heels and you feel a good stretch in your toes. Hold for thirty seconds to two minutes.

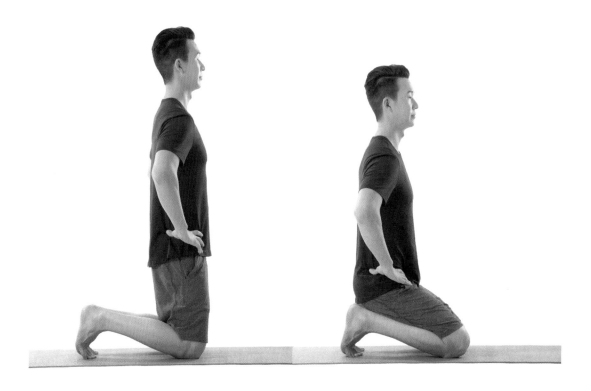

TOE STRETCH
(Standing)

Five toes = five things people rarely stretch. Of the five, the big toe is the most important from a functional standpoint, but the others team up to keep you standing, walking, and balancing. Don't forget these small but important body parts!

CUE

- To get a more intense stretch in the smaller toes, increase the angle of your foot.

TARGET AREAS

- Toes
- Feet
- Plantar fasciae

 HOW TO DO IT: Stand straight and tall, a few inches from a wall or block. Step forward with one foot, then angle it and place your toes up the wall or block. Place your hands on the wall (if using), then lean in until you feel a good stretch in your toes. Hold for thirty seconds to two minutes. Switch sides.

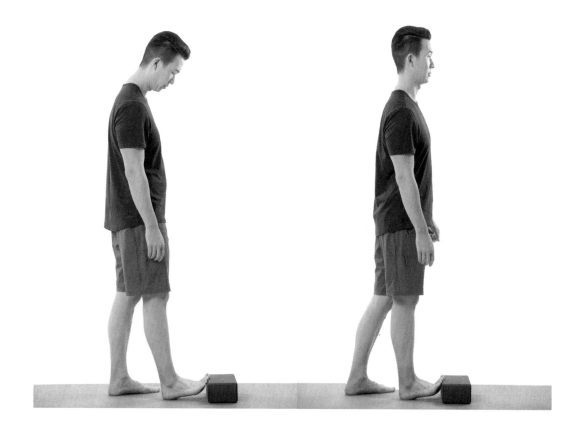

BIG TOE STRETCH
(Standing)

When I give my clients big toe stretches and mobility exercises, they give me a look that says, Are you serious?! I absolutely am! The big toe propels you forward when walking and can grip the ground to help you stay balanced. Kind of important, don't you think? So anytime someone gives you a funny look for stretching your big toe, drop this knowledge bomb on them. They may start big toe stretching, too.

CUES

- Other toes go to the side of the ball.
- To deepen the stretch, lean forward or take a small step forward while keeping working heel on the floor.

TARGET AREA

- Big toes

 HOW TO DO IT: Stand up straight and tall, and place your big toe on top of a tennis ball. Bend your knee slightly, and slide it forward to help your toe press down on the ball. Hold for thirty seconds to two minutes. Switch sides.

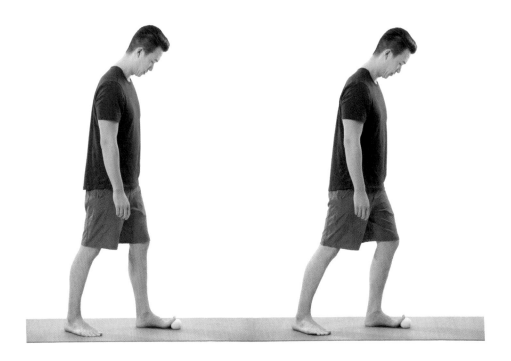

FOOT STEPOVER

If you like to take long walks or hikes, this stretch is for you. It stretches out the bottoms of the feet and ankles.

HOW TO DO IT: Place a rolled-up mat or towel on the floor. Standing straight and tall, step the front half of one foot onto the roll, keeping the heel on the floor. Take a small step forward with the other foot to stretch the raised foot. Do ten reps, holding each for two to five seconds. Switch sides.

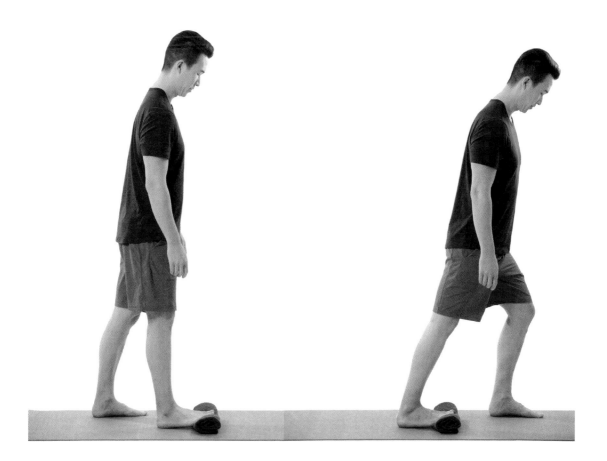

Ankles

Do you ever think about your ankles? Of course not. No one does! But here's why you should. The things that almost everybody does every day—like walking and squatting down—and things that some people do every day—like running and jumping—can be a lot tougher if your ankles are stiff. Inflexible ankles cause the body to overwork other areas to compensate for the lack of mobility. Imagine if you had blocks of concrete for ankles. The rest of your body would have to struggle to move to make up for those stiff joints. The knees in particular may torque in awkward ways, and that could then cause some wonky stuff to happen in your hips. You might end up with both knee *and* hip pain.

When talking about ankle mobility, you might think of flexing the ankle (pulling the foot toward you), but the ankles need to be able to move in the opposite direction (down), too. Likewise, they must be able to agilely shift from side to side—that will lower your risk of a twisted ankle. These stretches cover the full range of motion to keep your ankles flexible and allow your lower legs to move with greater ease.

WHAT ARE YOU IMPROVING?
Mobility in the ankle.

ADDED BENEFIT
Helps optimize performance in activities like walking, running, jumping, and squatting.

ANKLE MOBILITY EXERCISE (Half-Kneeling)

The more active you are, the more you need this ankle mobility exercise. Say you're on the basketball court and (as so often happens to basketball players) you turn your ankle. If it has mobility, you're going to walk away unscathed. If the muscle stays rigid, a sprain is the likely outcome. And you don't have to be a basketball player to have this same type of scenario play out. If you are walking and the sidewalk is uneven, a mobile ankle is going to keep you out of the ACE bandage section of the pharmacy. One way to judge if your ankle is stiff is to see how easy or hard it is to get your bent knee to shift out over your toes during this stretch. You may start out with little mobility, but the more you do it, the more your ankle is going to loosen up.

CUES

- Keep your heel on the floor.
- Don't allow your knee to cave in; make sure your knee stays over the middle or little toe.
- Place your hands on your knees for support.
- Point your hips forward.

TARGET AREAS

- Ankles
- Calves
- Achilles

HOW TO DO IT: Kneel on one leg with the toes tucked under, the other leg forward and bent at the knee, foot flat on the floor. Place your hands on your bent knee, and gently shift forward so your knee is over your toes. Hold for thirty seconds or two minutes. Switch sides.

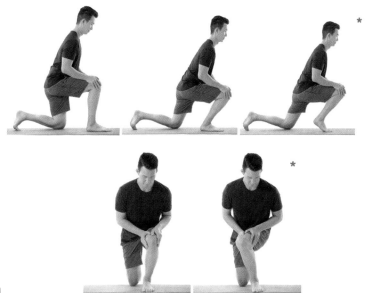

* IMPROPER FORM

ANKLE MOBILITY EXERCISE (Standing)

There's a good chance you've done something like this stretch before; when you hold the position, it's a common calf stretch for the back leg. The twist here is that you don't stay in a static pose. Instead, you add dynamic movement, which shifts the emphasis to stretching the front ankle rather than the rear calf.

 HOW TO DO IT: Stand straight and tall, hands on your hips. Step one foot back. Bend your front leg and lean in, sliding your knee over your toes until you feel a good stretch in your ankle. Straighten and bend your knee for ten reps. Switch sides.

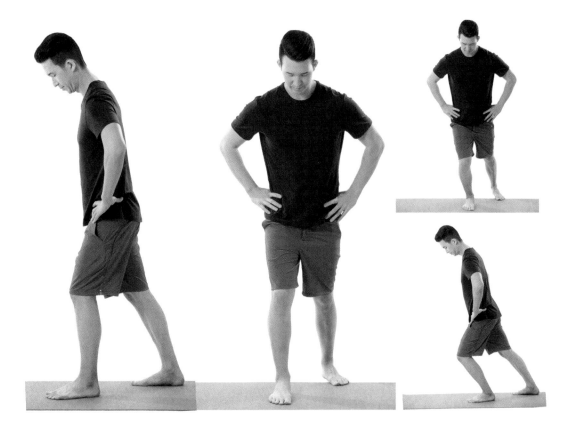

LEG SWINGS

Why are leg swings in the Lower Legs section of this book? Maybe you have seen this move before, used as a way to warm up the hips. In fact, it does both; it warms up the hips and, not so obviously, increases mobility in the ankles. The ankles need to not only dorsiflex and plantarflex (think pointing the feet toward you, then pointing them away from you), they also need to be able to move side to side. It's crucial in athletics but will also come in handy when you take that hike where the ground is bumpy with rocks and tree roots.

 HOW TO DO IT: Stand straight and tall, arms crossed in front of you. Swing one leg out to the side as far as you can comfortably go, then swing it across the other leg. Do ten reps. Switch sides.

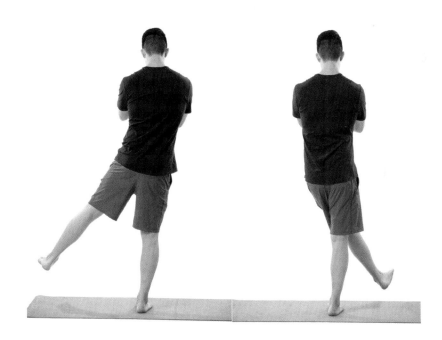

Calves

Now we're getting into some of the bigger muscles. The calf is actually made up of two muscles: the gastrocnemius and the soleus, both of which work hard when we walk or run. (If you want to impress your friends, here's how to pronounce gastrocnemius: gas-trok-NEE-me-us.) The footwear you choose can have a big impact on how your calves feel. High heels, in particular, put the calves in a shortened position, and that can lead to cramping. If high heels are part of your daily (or even occasional) wear, these stretches will be particularly important to add to your routine.

WHAT ARE YOU IMPROVING?
Lengthening of the calf muscles.

ADDED BENEFITS
Lowers risk of cramping; elongates the muscles shortened by heels or overworking.

CALF STRETCH
(Standing) (Gastrocnemius)

CUE

- Keep your back knee straight for the best gastrocnemius stretch.

TARGET AREAS

- Calves
- Ankles
- Achilles

This exercise is similar to the Toe Stretch Standing, but there is a crucial difference—in this stretch, you place more of the foot in the position. Holding the stretch homes in on the calf, which is exactly what you're going for here.

HOW TO DO IT: Stand straight and tall, hands on your hips. Place one leg behind you, flex your front foot, and place part of it on a block. (You can also use a wall to elevate your foot. Place hands flat on the wall for stability.) Keeping the front and back knee straight, raise your back heel until you feel a good stretch in the calf of your front leg. Hold for thirty seconds to two minutes. Switch sides.

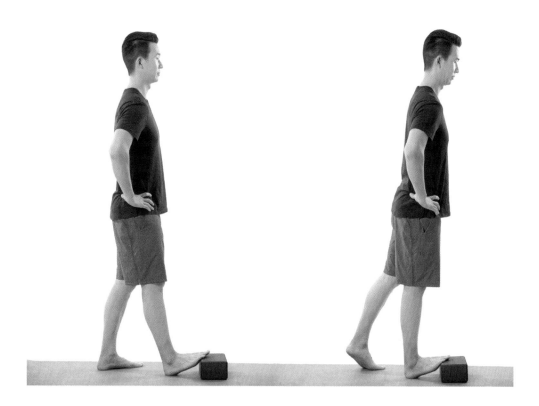

CALF STRETCH
(Standing) (Soleus)

The previous exercise targeted the superficial calf muscle. With this stretch, you're going to get into the muscle that lies beneath it, the soleus. The two work together to keep you on the move.

CUE
- Bend your front knee for the best soleus stretch.

TARGET AREAS
- Calves
- Ankles
- Achilles

HOW TO DO IT: Stand straight and tall, with your hands on your hips. Place one leg behind you, flex your front foot, and place part of it on a block. (You can also use a wall to elevate your foot. Place hands flat on the wall for stability.) Keeping your front knee bent, bend your back knee and lean forward until you feel a good stretch in the calf of your front leg. Hold for thirty seconds to two minutes. Switch sides.

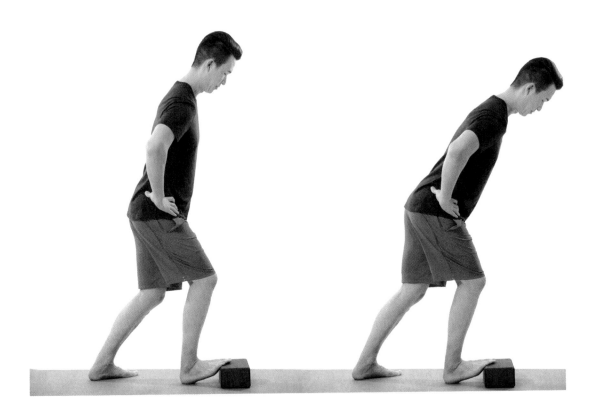

CALF STRETCH
(On All Fours)

If you have any tightness at all in your calves, you're going to really feel it when you do this stretch. Be sure to perform on both sides: You may even notice that one calf is tighter than the other. Make it your goal to get them equally supple.

CUES

- Keep your knees directly under your hips.
- Relax your neck.

TARGET AREAS

- Calves
- Ankles
- Toes
- Feet
- Plantar fasciae

HOW TO DO IT: Kneel on the floor, hands flat on the floor beneath your shoulders. Extend one leg behind you, toes on the floor and ankle flexed. Push into your hands, and move your body back until you feel the stretch in your calf. Hold for thirty seconds to two minutes. Switch sides.

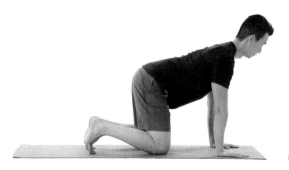
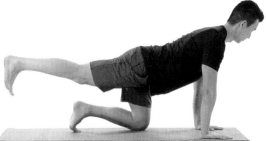
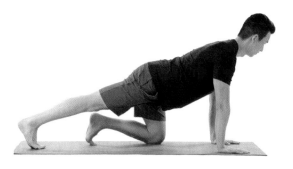
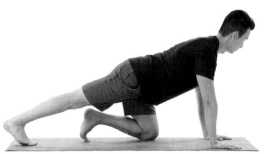

— 3 ——————————————————

STRETCHES FOR THE UPPER LEGS

The upper legs contain some of the biggest and strongest muscles in the body. These muscles, which include the hamstrings, quadriceps (quads), and adductor muscle group (inner thighs), do the brunt of the work when you move and suffer the most when you're stationary. These muscles also have outsize influence on other areas of the body. Tight quads, for instance, can pull the pelvis down, creating lower back pain. Tight hamstrings can tug at the hips, causing the same problem, and at the knee, sending pain to that region, as well. It's important, too, to keep these large muscles loose so you avoid injury; a muscle with little give is more prone to strains and tears.

Some of the stretches in this section may be familiar to you. Most people, if they learn to stretch at all, get to know some of the tried-and-true upper-leg stretches. Here you will learn how to do them properly and how to partner them with some stretches you probably have never done before. (Have you, for instance, ever heard of the Brettzel?) Familiar or not, the stretches are all very doable and will help counter the effects of anything you've been doing—from over-sitting to ambitious cycling—to shorten your body's biggest muscles.

The Quads

Cyclists and fans of indoor spinning generally know what it's like to have tight quads. The same is true for anyone else who participates in other thigh-centric activities (sprinting is one, rowing is another). If you don't do any of the above, you might not notice a lack of flexibility or feel much discomfort in the quads, but trust me, the four quad muscles that help you straighten your knee and move your leg forward need your attention.

WHAT ARE YOU IMPROVING?
Flexibility in the front of the thighs.

ADDED BENEFIT
Lessens risk of lower back pain.

QUAD STRETCH
(Standing)

Whenever I think of this stretch, I always envision someone warming up for a morning run. It's a classic, and for good reason. It does the job, it's easy, and it's straight to the point.

CUES

- Stand straight and tall, with your abs pulled in.
- Keep your knees close together.

TARGET AREA

- Quads

HOW TO DO IT: Stand on one leg, and if you need help with balance, stand with your side to a wall, and place your hand on the wall. Bend your outside leg, reach behind you, and grab your foot and pull it toward your butt until you feel a good stretch in the front of your thigh. Hold for thirty seconds to two minutes.

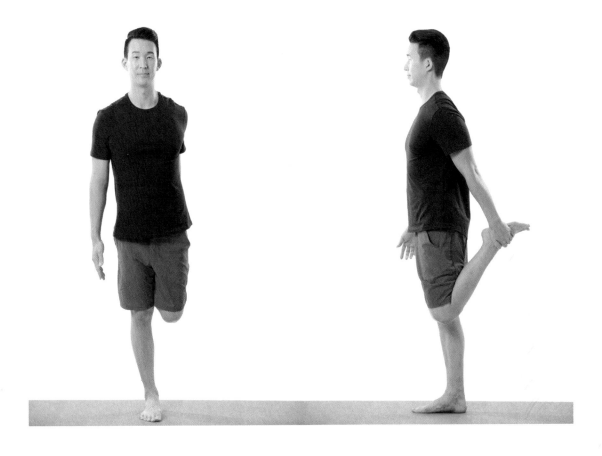

QUAD STRETCH
(Kneeling)

A lot of the time when people see this stretch, they worry it will be too hard on their knees. If you have knee problems, you may want to choose another quad stretch, or do this variation: Place a rolled-up towel or a foam roller between your butt and heels, which will lessen the bend in your knees. Then, instead of placing your hands on the floor behind you, do the exercise in front of a chair or couch, and rest your hands on the seat. This, too, will take some of the stress off the knees.

CUES

- Squeeze your butt, and push the hips forward to intensify the stretch.
- Your head stays in a neutral position.

TARGET AREAS

- Quads
- Hip flexors
- Ankles
- Shins

HOW TO DO IT: Sit on your heels, feet relaxed. Lean back and place your hands flat on the floor behind you until you feel a good stretch in your thighs. Hold for thirty seconds to two minutes.

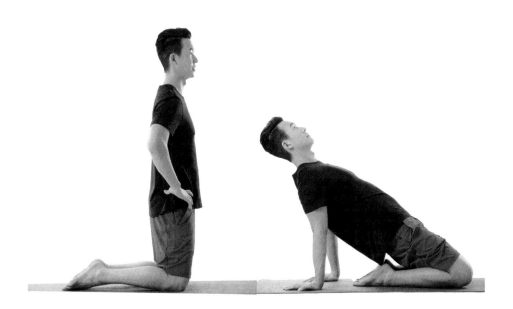

QUAD STRETCH
(On a Bench)

I'm showing this stretch on a workout bench, but it can also easily be done on the couch while you're watching TV. What could be better than that?! And, of course, it's effective. It really gets deep into the quads and hits the hip flexors as well.

CUE

- Squeeze your butt and abs.

TARGET AREAS

- Quads
- Hip flexors

HOW TO DO IT: Facing away from a bench, bend one knee, and place it on the floor in front of the bench. Place the other leg—bent at a 90-degree angle—and foot flat on the floor in front of you. Raise your upper body until you feel a good stretch in the front of your thigh. Hold for thirty seconds to two minutes. Switch sides.

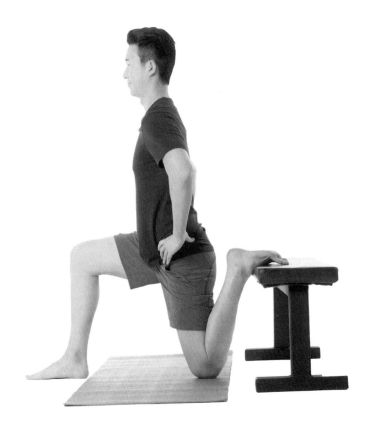

QUAD STRETCH
(On Your Side)

If you tried the Standing Quad Stretch and maybe felt a little wobbly, you may like this version better; it takes the balance component out of the stretch and is a good option until you feel comfortable doing it while standing.

CUES

- Keep your knees close together.
- Try not to arch your lower back.

TARGET AREAS

- Quads
- Hip flexors

 HOW TO DO IT: Lie on your side, rest your head in your hand, and bend your top leg back toward your butt. Grab the ankle and pull until you feel a good stretch in the front of your thigh. Hold for thirty seconds to two minutes. Switch sides.

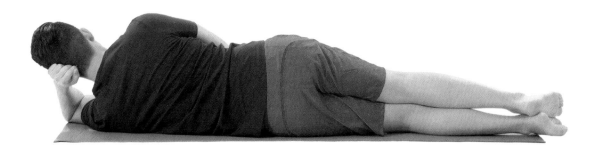

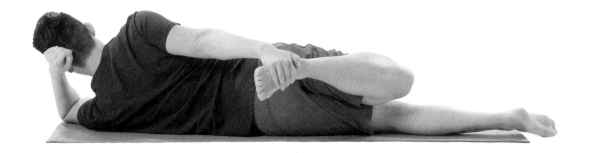

Hamstrings and Inner Thighs

Tight hamstrings are the curse of the modern world! Maybe that's a little extreme, but most people feel like they have tight hamstrings. These stretches address not only the hamstrings but the adductor (inner thigh) muscles. You really want these muscles to be agile. What if, for instance, you need to hop over a big puddle on the sidewalk? What if you're taking a cardio class at the gym that requires some vigorous side-to-side or back-to-front moves? If you're literally hamstrung, plus your inner thigh muscles have little give, you'll be at a much greater risk of injury.

WHAT ARE YOU IMPROVING?
Flexibility in the backs of the thighs and inner thighs.

ADDED BENEFITS
Increases ease of movement while walking or running; provides relief in the lower back due to tight muscles pulling on the pelvis.

WIDE-LEGGED HAMSTRING STRETCH

I've been doing this stretch for what feels like forever (or at least since elementary school gym class). I still do it all the time because it stretches out the hamstrings, hits the inner thighs, and because it's a great way to just let tension go. Hinge over those legs, and just let it all hang out!

CUES

- A short foam roller can fill in for a block.
- Bend your knees slightly to avoid rounding or arching your back.

TARGET AREAS

- Hamstrings
- Inner thighs

HOW TO DO IT: Standing straight and tall, separate your legs wide (about double shoulder-width apart), toes pointing forward. Hinge forward, and place your hands on the floor. If you struggle with this or prefer to keep your back straighter, hold one or more yoga blocks and then hinge forward until the block reaches the floor. This will allow you to keep your back straight. You should feel a good stretch in the backs of your legs. Hold for thirty seconds to two minutes.

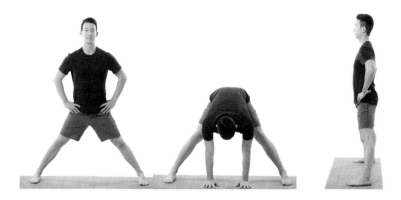

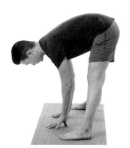

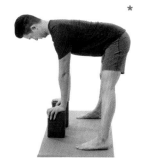

*

* VARIATION

WIDE-LEGGED HAMSTRING TO ONE SIDE STRETCH

CUE

- Push your hips back.

TARGET AREAS

- Hamstrings
- Inner thighs

This stretch begins with a pause: You hinge forward and rest your hands on the floor or on blocks or books. I think it's a good way to start; it gives you a nice stretch in both legs before you elongate them individually. However, if you don't want to bother with blocks or books (but can't touch the floor), just let your arms hang down for a few seconds and then continue on with the rest of the exercise.

HOW TO DO IT: Separate your legs wide (about double shoulder-width apart), toes pointing forward. Hinge forward and, if possible, touch the floor. (If you can't touch the floor, rest your hands on yoga blocks or upright books.) Walk your hands over to one foot (or shin) until you feel a good stretch in the back of your leg. Hold for thirty seconds to two minutes. Switch sides.

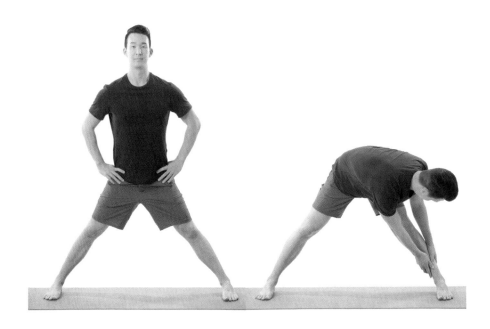

LEG DROPS WITH A TOWEL

You can also do this dynamic stretch with a belt or exercise band—anything that you can loop around the bottom of your foot.

- Keep your legs straight or slightly bent at the knee.
- Head, shoulders, and back stay flat on the floor.

TARGET AREA

- Hamstrings

 HOW TO DO IT: Lie on your back. Raise one leg to 90 degrees, and loop a towel around the bottom of your foot; hold the towel ends with both hands. Keeping your back flat, raise your other leg up to the same height. Keeping a good grip on the towel, lower the non-looped leg to the floor. Do ten reps. Switch sides.

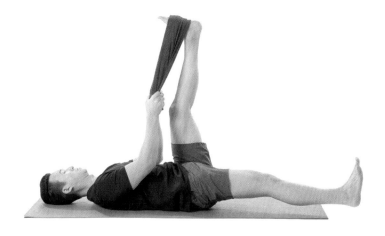

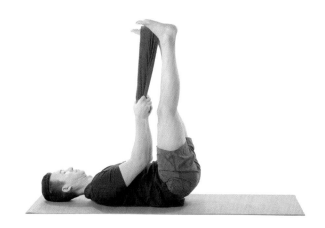

MODIFIED HAMSTRING STRETCH (Standing)

Simple and classic, this stretch gets deep into the hamstrings.

CUES

- Keep your back fairly flat.
- Slide your hips back farther to intensify the stretch.

TARGET AREA

- Hamstrings

HOW TO DO IT: Stand straight and tall, feet hip-width apart. Bring one leg forward about a foot, foot flat on the floor, leg straight. Keeping your back straight and abs engaged, bend the opposite knee, and slide your hips back as if sitting. Place both hands on your hips for support. Hold for thirty seconds to two minutes. Switch sides.

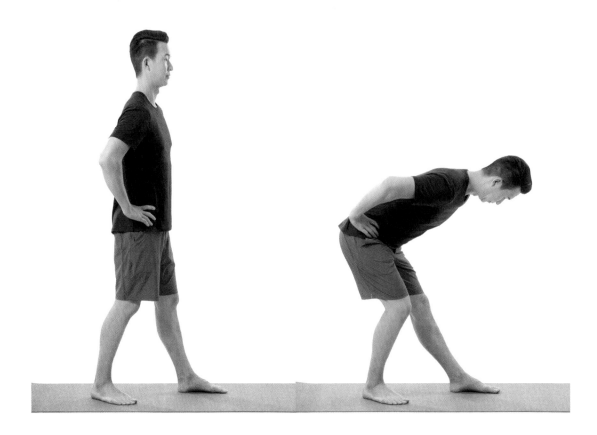

GROIN STRETCH
(Half-Kneeling)

The groin area contains a type of muscle called adductors. Awkward and sudden movements (common in sports like hockey, soccer, and football) can be hard on these muscles, causing groin strain. Keeping them supple will help you avoid injury and just make movement easier all around.

CUES

- Make sure your knee stays over the middle or little toe.
- Shoulders and hips should remain facing forward.

TARGET AREA

- Groin

 HOW TO DO IT: Kneel on one leg, the other leg forward and bent at the knee, foot flat on the floor. Still bent, swing the forward leg out to the side, toes pointed out at a 90-degree angle. Keeping your upper body upright and facing forward, shift to the side and allow your front knee to move over your toes until you feel a good stretch in your inner thigh and groin. Hold for thirty seconds to two minutes. Switch sides.

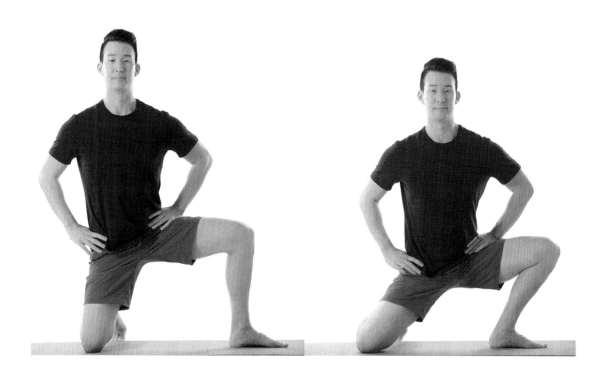

GROIN ROCKING STRETCH

Will this rocking groin move rock your world?
I hope so! At the very least, it's going to give you
an incredible stretch in this hard-to-reach area.

CUE

- Shoulders and hips should remain facing forward.

TARGET AREA

- Groin

HOW TO DO IT: Get down on all fours, then swing one leg out to the side, keeping it straight. Keeping your back straight, shift your hips back toward your back foot until you feel a good stretch in your inner thigh and groin. Hold for thirty seconds to two minutes. Switch sides.

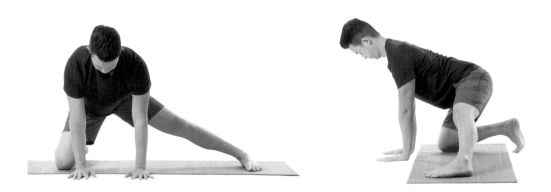

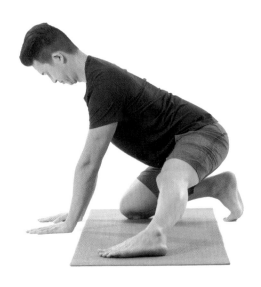

GROIN STRETCH WITH SIDE BEND

This is a classic two-for-the-price-of-one stretch. It's main focus is the groin—and believe me, you will feel it when you move into position—but it also gives you a nice side stretch, hitting the lats and the QL (quadratus lumborum), a muscle I'll tell you more about in chapter 5.

CUE

- Don't let your upper body collapse into the stretch.

TARGET AREAS

- Groin
- Lats
- Quadratus lumborum (QL)

HOW TO DO IT: Kneel with one leg out to the side, heel on the floor, your upper body straight and tall. Raise the arm opposite the extended leg, point the other arm down between your legs, and bend your upper body to the side. Hold for thirty seconds to two minutes. Switch sides.

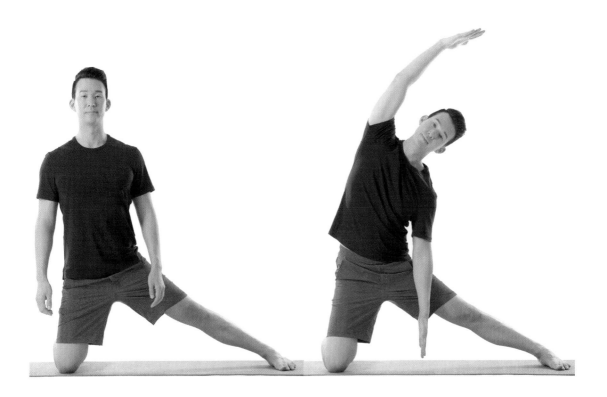

STANDING HAMSTRING STRETCH ON A BENCH

This exercise calls for something to prop your legs on. I'm using a bench, but you can use the seat of a chair, a railing, or anything else that gets your legs up at slightly lower than or at hip height.

CUES

- The higher your leg, the more intense the stretch.
- Optional: Reach your arms toward your feet, if possible, grabbing hold of your toes.
- Straighten your knee to get a more intense stretch.

TARGET AREA

- Hamstrings

 HOW TO DO IT: Prop one leg on a bench, knee slightly bent. Hinge at the hips, and reach your upper body over your raised leg until you feel a good stretch in the back of your leg. Hold for thirty seconds to two minutes. Switch sides. If you bend your knee, you'll feel the stretch in your hamstrings more.

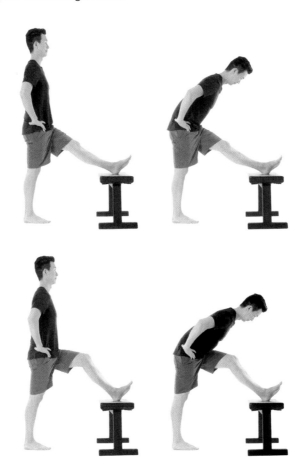

HAMSTRING 90/90 STRETCH

The beauty of this stretch is that you get to lie back and relax while doing it. It not only does the trick in terms of lengthening the hamstrings, it also can help ease sciatica symptoms.

CUE

- Inactive leg stays straight.

TARGET AREA

- Hamstrings

HOW TO DO IT: Lie faceup on the floor. Bring one knee to hip level, bent at a 90-degree angle. Keep the other leg straight on the floor. Clasp your hands lightly around the thigh of your raised leg, and kick up the lower part of the leg, straightening it as much as comfortably possible. Do ten reps. Switch sides.

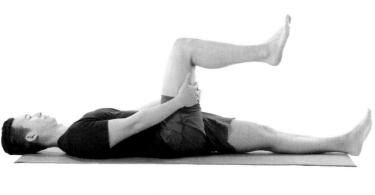

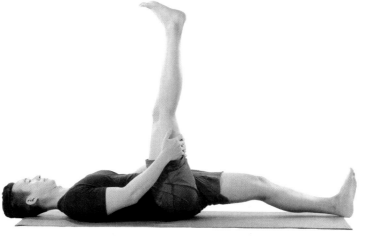

LAZY GROIN STRETCH

It's a little tricky getting up into this position, but once you master it, I think you'll really enjoy it. For the stretch, you open your legs wide, but it's also nice to bring your legs together and just relax in the position for a while. As long as you're there, why not?

CUES

- Your heels rest on the wall.
- Enjoy! You don't have to do anything to get a stretch.

TARGET AREA

- Inner thighs

HOW TO DO IT: Lie with your upper body on the floor, faceup, as you move your butt as close to a wall as possible and swing your legs up the wall. Spread your legs wide until you feel a good stretch in your groin. Hold for thirty seconds to two minutes.

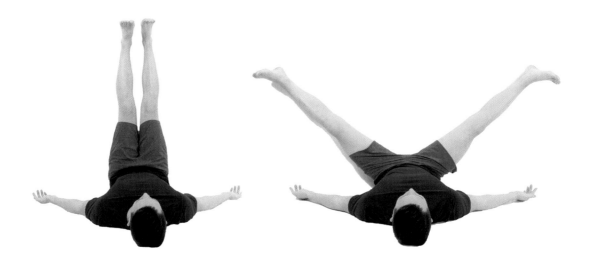

BUTTERFLY STRETCH

Another one of those stretches that never goes out of style—I remember doing it back in gym class. A simple seated stretch that hits the groin.

CUE

- To increase the stretch, bend your elbows and gently push down on your knees.

TARGET AREA

- Groin

 HOW TO DO IT: Sit down on the floor, bend your knees, and bring the soles of your feet together. (I like to place my hands on my feet as if holding them together.) Sit up straight and tall, then slowly let your knees fall toward the floor until you feel a good stretch in your groin. Hold for thirty seconds to two minutes.

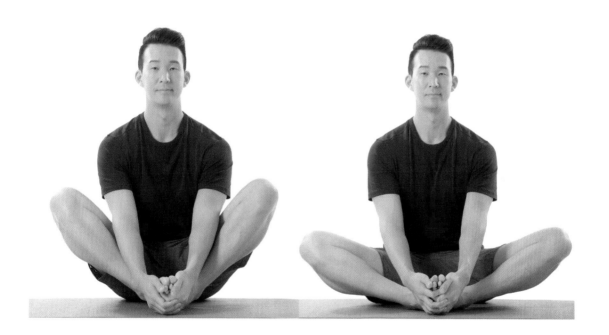

FROG POSE

You might get some weird looks if you do this move in public, but it's so good for your hips and groin that it's worth it! Shift back into the stretch and feel your body melt.

CUES

- The wider apart your knees, the deeper the stretch.
- To intensify the stretch even more, bring your forearms down to the floor in front of you.

TARGET AREA

- Inner thighs

 HOW TO DO IT: Kneel on the floor with your knees wide, feet facing outward, hands beneath your shoulders. Keeping your upper body straight, shift back toward your feet until you feel a good stretch in your thighs and groin. Hold for thirty seconds to two minutes.

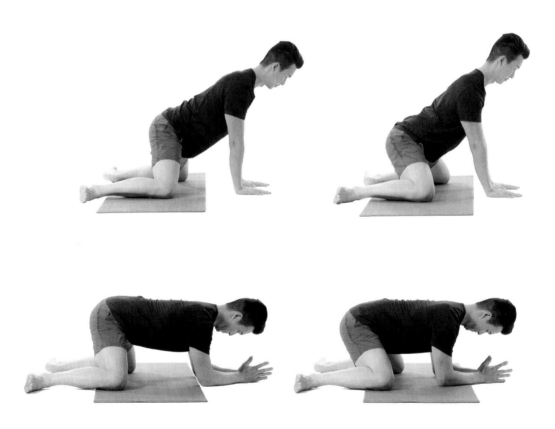

THE BRETTZEL

This stretch got its name from the person who popularized it, a guy named Brett Jones, as well as its twisty, pretzel-like shape.

CUES

- The more flexible you are, the closer your shoulder will get to the floor.
- A pillow is optional, but it is nice to have some support.

TARGET AREAS

- Hip flexors
- Quads
- T-spine

HOW TO DO IT: Lie on your side with your head on a pillow (if desired). Bend your top leg so the knee is at hip level, and hold your thigh with your hand. Bend your bottom leg, and catch the foot with your other hand. Rotate your body to drop your shoulder and the foot you're holding toward the floor until you feel a good stretch in the thigh. Hold for thirty seconds to two minutes. Switch sides.

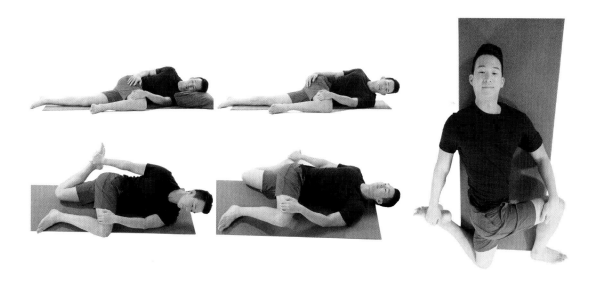

— 4

STRETCHES FOR THE HIPS AND GLUTES

Would you believe your butt is one of the strongest muscles in the body? The glutes (as the butt is sometimes referred to, short for gluteus maximus, one of the muscles in the butt) and their neighbors, the hip flexors and hip rotators, need to have a good range of motion and be strong for the body to function properly. When they don't, so many things can go wrong, from knee and/or hip pain to sciatica. The enemy of hip and glute flexibility is, not surprisingly, sitting. Staying in the seated position for hours on end makes these muscles lazy; they don't want to move, and as a result, they can feel somewhat frozen.

Most of the time, we move in one plane—forward and back, but when we need to rotate, we call on the hip and glute muscles. If they're not supple and fit, your range of motion will be poor, which means any rotation-dependent activity—like tennis or golf or simply reaching across your body to grab something off a shelf—will not go as well as it could.

This chapter has exercises that ease tightness and promote mobility in the hips and butt. On page 72, you'll also find a move that may help ease the pain of sciatica, a fiery pain that runs down the leg.

Hips and Glutes

How breezily you can walk. Lower back pain. The effectiveness of your weight training program. What do these three things have in common? Hip flexor flexibility. Hip flexors connect the top of the leg to the lower back and hip. By helping you bend your knees and bend at the waist, they affect the overall mobility of your body. If you're slow or don't seem to be getting the most out of your lower-body weight training, tight hip flexors might be to blame. Since the hip muscles connect to the butt, I've coupled hip flexor stretches with stretches for the glutes. All these muscles work together, so they need equal amounts of care.

WHAT ARE YOU IMPROVING?
Flexibility in the hips and butt.

ADDED BENEFITS
Improves back pain and optimizes exercise that requires hip extension such as walking, running, soccer, and tennis.

HIP FLEXOR STRETCH
(Half-Kneeling)

Stretching doesn't get much simpler than this. You don't need to twist yourself into a knot to achieve the main objective here: muscles that are suppler and allow you to move easily in all the directions you need to.

CUES

- Don't let your back arch.
- Keep your upper body upright and in the same plane as your hips.

TARGET AREA

- Hip flexors

HOW TO DO IT: Kneel on one leg, the other leg forward and bent at the knee, foot flat on the floor. With your upper body straight and tall, arms crossed in front of you, tighten your butt and abs, and shift forward toward your toes until you feel a good stretch in your hip. Hold for thirty seconds to two minutes. Switch sides.

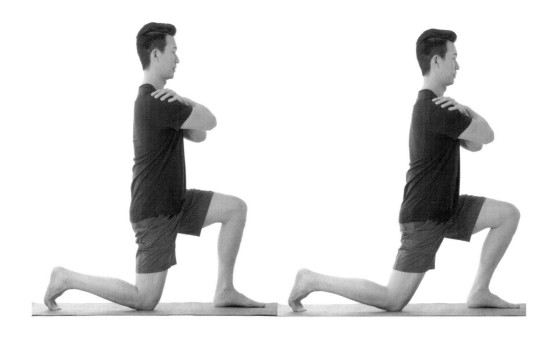

THREE-WAY HIP STRETCH

I'm a big fan of moving in multiple directions when stretching because our bodies also move in multiple directions during daily life. This hip stretch starts by moving forward, then transitions to the side in two different ways. It hits all the hip's ranges of motion and also provides a deep groin stretch.

CUES

- Keep your hips facing forward.
- Make sure your knee stays over the middle or little toe.

TARGET AREAS

- Hip flexors
- Groin

HOW TO DO IT: Kneel on one leg with your foot relaxed, the other leg forward and bent at the knee, foot flat on the floor. Part 1: Tighten your butt and abs, and, keeping your upper body upright, shift forward so your knee moves over your toes and you feel a good stretch in the front of your hip. Hold for thirty seconds to two minutes. Part 2: Move back to an upright position, then swing your front leg to the side at about a 45-degree angle, knee still bent and foot flat on the floor. With your body upright, shift forward so your knee moves over your toes and you feel a good stretch in your hip and groin. Hold for thirty seconds to two minutes. Part 3: Open up the leg farther to the side, to about a 90-degree angle, then with your hips facing forward, shift your upper body over your knee so the knee moves over your toes and you feel a good stretch in the groin. Hold for thirty seconds to two minutes. Switch sides.

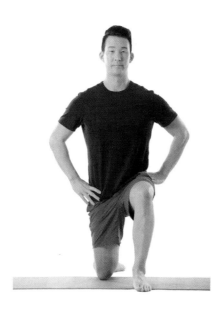

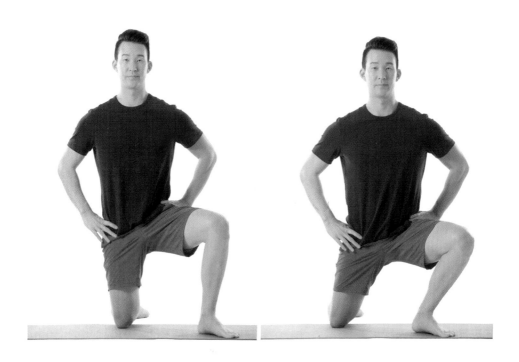

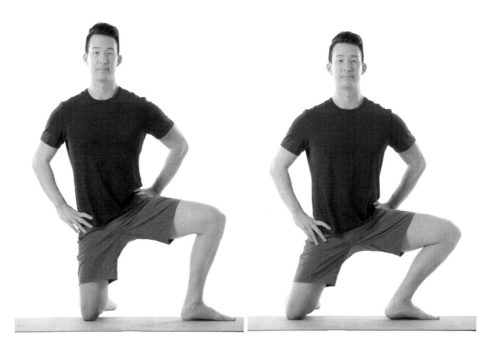

90/90 STRETCH FOR HIP EXTERNAL AND INTERNAL ROTATION

CUES

- Keep your back straight as you lean forward.
- Brace yourself with your hands.

TARGET AREA

- Hips

We spend a lot of time stretching the fronts and backs of our bodies, but don't forget that we humans rotate. The 90/90 position has become a favorite of mine in the past few years because it is about as efficient an exercise as you can get. With this one simple stretch, you'll work all the ways the hip can rotate.

HOW TO DO IT: Sit on the floor with one leg in front of you, knee bent at a 90-degree angle, and the other leg behind you, knee also bent at a 90-degree angle. Flex both feet, and sit up straight and tall. Lean forward until you feel a good stretch in the back of your hip. Hold for thirty seconds to two minutes. Place your arms out in front of you, and rotate toward the back foot until you feel a good stretch in the front of your hip. Hold for thirty seconds to two minutes. Switch sides.

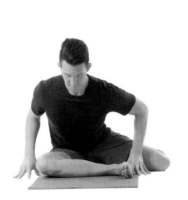
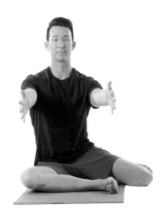
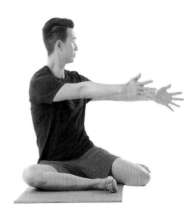

90/90 STRETCH WITH SIDE BEND

It's rare that you hit only one muscle group when you stretch. This exercise, while primarily for the hips, also stretches the QL, which can help with lower back pain (more on this in chapter 5).

CUE

- If placing your forearm on the floor is difficult, prop yourself up on your hand instead.

TARGET AREAS

- Hips
- Lats
- QL

HOW TO DO IT: Sit on the floor with one leg in front of you, knee bent at a 90-degree angle, and the other leg behind you, knee also bent at a 90-degree angle. Flex both feet, and sit up straight and tall. Drop the arm next to your front leg to the floor and rest on your forearm. Raise the other arm overhead and stretch to the side. Hold for thirty seconds to two minutes. Switch sides.

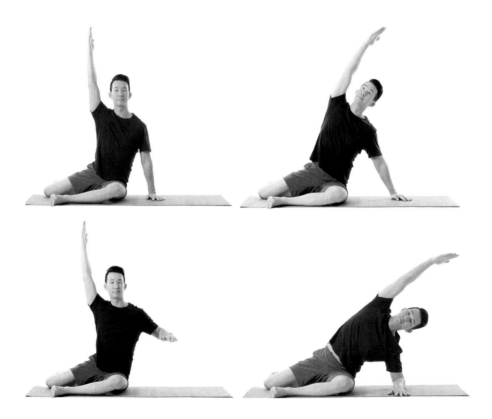

90/90 STRETCH WITH LEAN BACK

On some days (and even at different times of day), you will undoubtedly feel more limber than on others. As you do this and other stretches, try to take account of how flexible you feel and compare it to other times. Then ask yourself why. Did you sit more and move less on a tight day? Does your body move more easily at the end of the day than in the morning? Did your workout make you tighter or looser? Stretching doesn't just improve your body; it helps you get to know it better.

HOW TO DO IT: Sit on the floor with one leg in front of you, knee bent at a 90-degree angle, and the other leg behind you, knee also bent at a 90-degree angle. Place your hands on the floor behind you, and lean back until you feel a good stretch in the front of your hip. Hold for thirty seconds to two minutes. Switch sides.

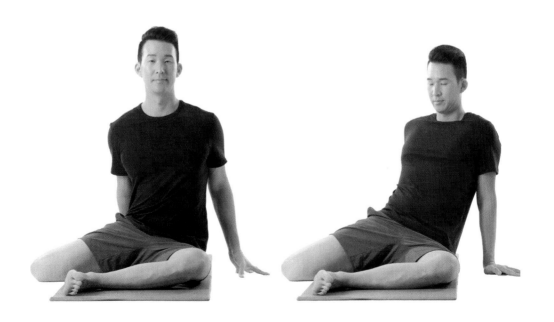

90/90 MOVING STRETCH

CUES

- Back stays loose but not rounded.
- Move at a moderate pace.

TARGET AREA

- Hips

This dynamic stretch is so rhythmic, it should be set to music! Holding your arms out in front of you calls for balance; if it's too difficult, try the next variation 90/90 Moving Stretch with Support.

HOW TO DO IT: Sit with your legs open wide, knees bent, feet flexed, and heels resting on the floor. Place your arms out in front of you at shoulder height. Twist to one side, dropping your knees down to the floor as you go. Hold for two to five seconds, then swing your knees to the other side. Do ten reps, alternating side to side.

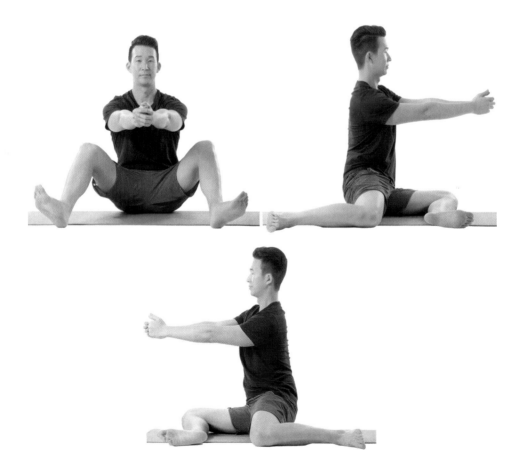

90/90 MOVING STRETCH WITH SUPPORT

CUE

- Move at a moderate pace.

TARGET AREA

- Hips

Like the version of this exercise without support, this dynamic stretch calls for swinging your knees back and forth. If they don't touch the floor, don't worry; just drop them as low as they can comfortably go.

 HOW TO DO IT: Sit with your legs open wide, knees bent, feet flexed, and heels resting on the floor. Place your arms behind you, hands flat on the floor. Twist to one side, dropping your knees down to the floor as you go. Hold for two to five seconds, then swing your knees to the other side. Do ten reps, alternating side to side.

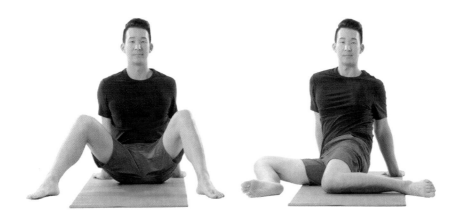

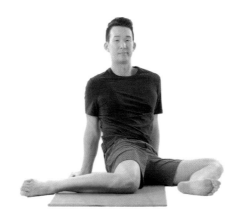

MODIFIED LIZARD POSE

Lizard Pose takes the standard hip flexor stretch to the next level. I first tried this in a yoga class and knew immediately that it would become a staple stretch in my routine.

CUE

- For a more intense stretch, bring your forearms to the floor.

TARGET AREA

- Hip flexors

 HOW TO DO IT: From a push-up position, bring one leg forward, and place your foot next to your hand. Drop your hip down until you feel a good stretch in the hip and groin. Hold for thirty seconds to two minutes. Switch sides.

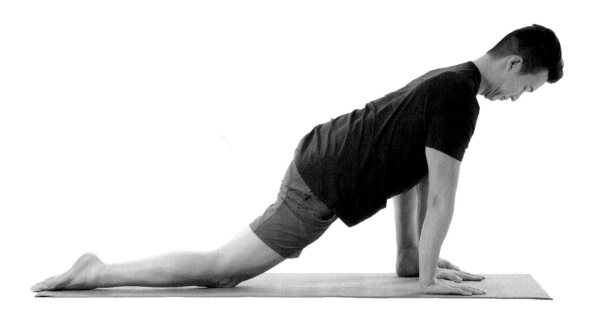

PIGEON POSE

There's a good reason why this is one of most popular stretches around. It's a great way to target the external rotators of the hip and the piriformis, a small muscle located deep in the butt. Sometimes the piriformis can get a little tight and affect the sciatic nerve. When that's the case, this move can help.

CUES

- Open or close the angle of your bent leg depending on your flexibility.
- Resting on your forearms gives the deepest stretch.
- Your neck stays relaxed, face toward the floor.

TARGET AREA

- Hips

HOW TO DO IT: From a push-up position, bring one leg forward and drop it to the floor, knee bent. If you're very flexible, your leg should be at a 90-degree angle with your shin parallel to your shoulders. If you're less flexible, allow your lower leg to bend in toward your groin at a 45-degree angle or less. Stretch the back leg behind you, and with your chest out, lower your upper body and bring it to rest on your forearms. If that's too intense, stay up on your hands. Hold for thirty seconds to two minutes. Switch sides.

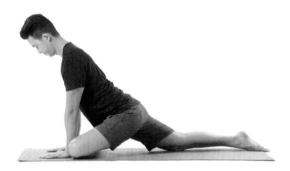

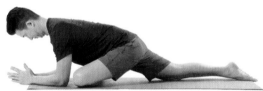

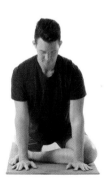

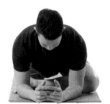

PIGEON POSE ON A BENCH

Pigeon Pose is a very intense exercise, but you can make it less so by using a table or, as I do here, a bench. You will still get a profound stretch and, if you like, can work your way up to Pigeon Pose on the floor. Either way, you're going to be doing your hips a favor.

CUES

- Open or close the angle of your bent leg depending on your flexibility.
- Your neck stays relaxed, face toward the bench.

TARGET AREA

- Hips

 HOW TO DO IT: Stand in front of a table or bench. Place one leg on the table, knee bent at a 90-degree angle. Keeping your upper body straight and tall, hinge forward over the bent leg. Hold for thirty seconds to two minutes. Switch sides.

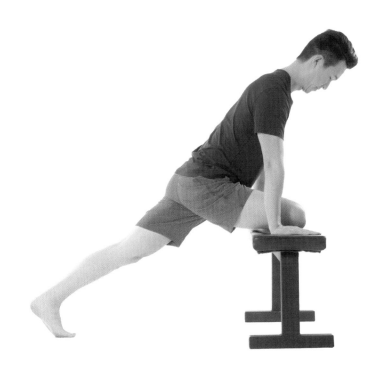

HIP FLEXOR STRETCH ON A BENCH

Long days spent sitting are the enemy of the hip flexors. This is a great stretch to do when you come home from work, a way to shake off the cobwebs that accumulate during a deskbound day.

CUES

- Concentrate on the crease where your hip meets your leg.
- Your upper body stays lifted.

TARGET AREA

- Hip flexors

HOW TO DO IT: Stand with your side to a table or bench, and place your inside leg on top, foot hanging off. Bend the other leg into a high lunging position. With your hands on the table in front of you, tighten your butt and abs, lean forward, and gently drive your hip down toward the table until you feel a good stretch in the front of the hip. Hold for thirty seconds to two minutes. Switch sides.

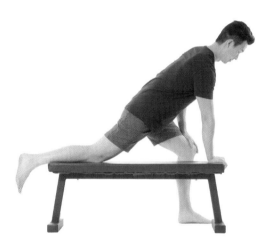
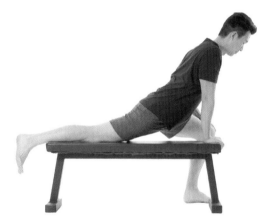

TACTICAL FROG

This stretch rivals its partner, the Frog Pose, in awkwardness—and efficiency. It's called "tactical" because it gets into those hips and groin with military precision!

CUE

- Your spine stays neutral.

TARGET AREAS

- Hips
- Groin

 HOW TO DO IT: Get down on your hands and knees, then slide your knees wide out to the side and point your toes out. In one smooth move, slide your butt back toward your feet, then shift forward and, as you go, bring one of your feet toward the ceiling, keeping your knee on the floor. Switch sides. Do ten reps, alternating side to side.

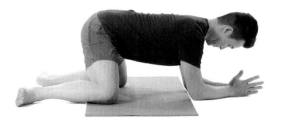 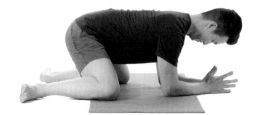

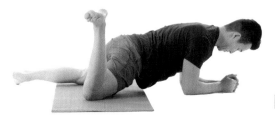 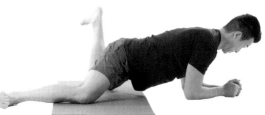

THE BRETTZEL 2.0

Again, hats off to Brett Jones, who came up with this and the original Brettzel moves. Don't be put off by its twisty, turny, and somewhat strange-looking positioning; it's quite easy to do, and the payoff is big.

CUES

- Avoid hunching.
- Your arms stay straight.

TARGET AREAS

- Hips
- T-spine

HOW TO DO IT: Sit on the floor with one leg in front of you, knee bent at a 90-degree angle, and the other leg behind you, that knee also bent at a 90-degree angle. Flex both feet, and sit up straight and tall. Place your hand on the floor next to your front knee. Take the other hand and place it, palm up, under the hand next to your front knee. Staying tall, with your chest out, drop your shoulder toward your front foot until you feel a good stretch in your hip. Hold for thirty seconds to two minutes. Switch sides.

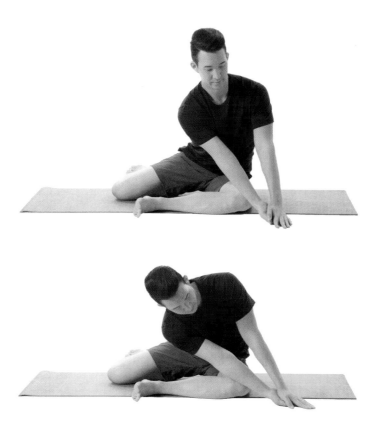

FIGURE-FOUR SUPPORTED STRETCH

Why so many variations on the Figure-Four Stretch? One is not necessarily better than the other, but it's just that one might suit your particular body best. It's great to have options in everything, and that includes stretching.

CUES

- To deepen the stretch, pull the foot closer to your butt.
- To ease up, slide the foot away from your butt.

TARGET AREA

- Hips

HOW TO DO IT: Sit down on the floor with your legs outstretched. Lean back slightly, and place your arms behind you, hands flat on the floor to support your weight. Place the ankle of one leg just above the knee of the other. Bend the outstretched leg, and slide it toward your upper body until you feel a good stretch in your hip. Hold for thirty seconds to two minutes. Switch sides.

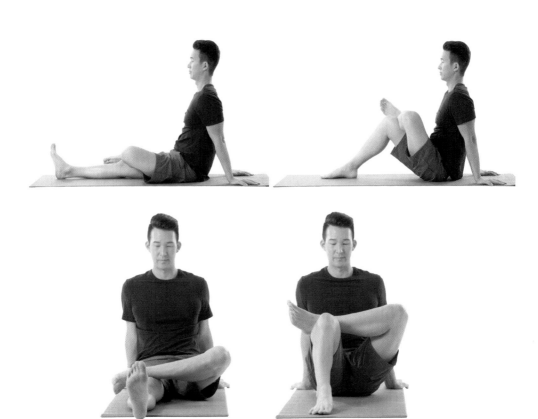

FIGURE-FOUR LYING-DOWN STRETCH

This is essentially the same stretch as the Figure-Four performed supported, but since you do it lying down, it fits in nicely with any mat work you're doing at the gym. It can also be done in bed right when you wake up in the morning to get your body going. It's like coffee for the hips!

CUE

- The harder you pull your legs in toward your chest, the intenser the stretch.

TARGET AREA

- Hips

 HOW TO DO IT: Lie on the floor faceup, knees bent, feet flat. Cross one leg over the other, and rest your ankle on your knee, foot flexed. Raise your bottom leg toward your chest, and clasp your hands beneath your knee or around the back of your thigh and gently pull your legs in closer. Hold for thirty seconds to two minutes. Switch sides.

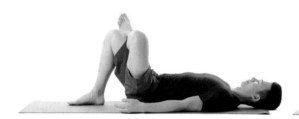

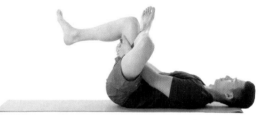

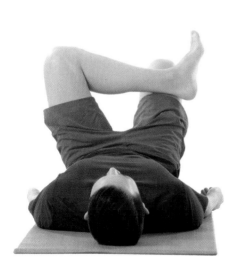

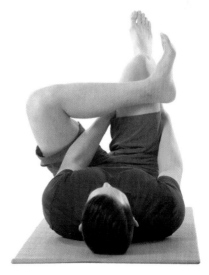

EASING SCIATICA

Sciatica is the kind of problem that can be confusing. You feel pain down your leg, but when you try massaging the achiness away, it doesn't feel soothing the way it normally does when you rub a sore muscle. That's because the pain really isn't coming from the muscle; it's nerve related. Sciatica occurs when nerves become entrapped or compressed. The glute stretches in this chapter can help take the pressure off the nerve and relieve the pain. (Other good stretches for sciatica: Pigeon Pose [page 65] and Hamstring 90/90 Stretch [page 49].)

The exercise below is a different type of stretch; it actually stretches the affected nerves instead of the muscles surrounding them. At first glance, it will seem to have nothing to do with anything going on in your legs, but give it a try. It may very well help give you some relief.

SCIATIC NERVE GLIDE

Sit on a bench or table. Extend one leg, and flex the foot as you bend your neck and tilt your head back. Hold for a second. Lower your leg as you bend your neck forward and tuck your chin. Do ten to fifteen reps, alternating forward and backward movements. Switch sides.

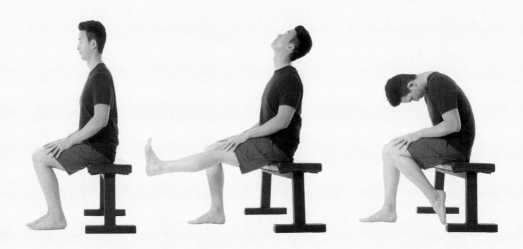

— 5 —————————————————

STRETCHES FOR THE LOWER BACK

The best stretches for the lower back are stretches for other parts of the body. That's probably not something you were expecting, but when you think about it, it makes sense; when the glutes, quads, and hip flexors are tight, they tug on the lower back and hips, making them ache or even throwing them completely out of whack. The culprit behind a tight lower back can also be the mid- or upper back—when those spots are stiff, the low back compensates for the lack of movement above.

You can find stretches for those lower back–adjacent muscles in separate chapters, and they will undoubtedly help loosen up the area. But I also have something lower back–specific for you here. There is a critical muscle in the lower back that attaches from the top of the pelvis to the last rib and can be a source of trouble. It's called the quadratus lumborum, or QL for short. The QL helps you bend to the side and is also involved in walking. When other muscles in the area are inflexible, they can cause the QL to tighten up. If it's rigid, you may see your hip hike up on one side. In fact, many people think they have one leg that's shorter than the other, only to discover it's just the QL pulling on the hip and causing a body imbalance.

I am cautious about recommending stretches as a cure for pain relief. But in some people, QL stretches actually can soothe the lower back. Give them a try, gently so as not to cause yourself more pain. If you don't have pain, the QL stretches can help keep your back healthy.

The stretches in this chapter also hit the spinal erectors. Spinal erectors are the muscles that run along the spine from the lower back all the way up to the back of your head. Essentially, they help hold up your back.

QL

If you have ever had a massage, you know the difference between light kneading and a deep-tissue rubdown. Think of these QL stretches as the deep-tissue type of stretching; they get at an area of the body that other stretches miss. You can also help keep this muscle in good working order by strengthening it. The core exercises in chapter 10 are good companions for the stretches here.

WHAT ARE YOU IMPROVING?
Flexibility in the side muscles.

ADDED BENEFITS
Lessens lower back pain and increases mobility in the side of your body (helpful for things like serving in tennis and reaching up and across to grab something off a shelf).

CHILD'S POSE

In yoga, Child's Pose is considered a rest position. But while you're doing all that resting, you are also getting an incredible stretch in your lower back. This stretch can be done on the floor or on a softer surface, like a bed. I recommend doing it often.

CUES

- Widen your legs as much as you'd like; this is a personal choice.
- As you loosen up, shimmy your hands forward for a more intense stretch.

TARGET AREA

- Lats

 HOW TO DO IT: Sit back on your heels, toes touching, knees apart. Lower your upper body between your knees, stretch your arms forward, and place your forehead on or near the floor. You should feel a good stretch in your back. Hold for thirty seconds to two minutes.

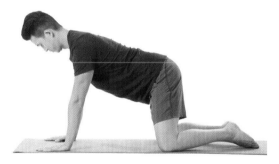
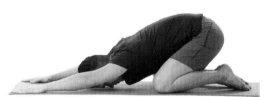
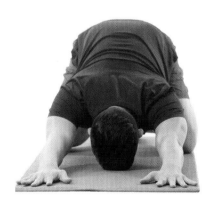

DYNAMIC CHILD'S POSE

By building movement into the pose, this move takes Child's Pose to a whole new level. As you go, you are not only elongating the back but "greasing the wheels" of the hip joints, helping to keep them from getting tight and creaky.

CUE

- Widen your legs as much as you'd like; this is a personal choice.

TARGET AREAS

- Low back
- Lats
- Spinal erectors

 HOW TO DO IT: Sit back on your heels, toes touching, knees apart. Lower your upper body between your knees, stretch your arms forward, and place your forehead on or near the floor. Lift your head and slide forward to an all-fours position, then drive your hips back into Child's Pose. Do ten reps.

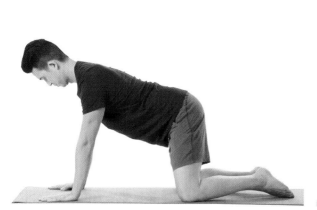
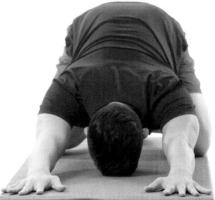
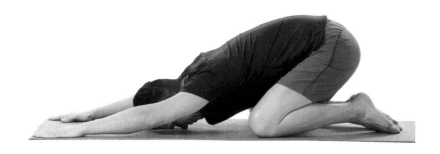

MODIFIED HURDLER STRETCH WITH SIDE BEND

CUE

- Maintain length in the upper body.

TARGET AREAS

- Low back
- Lats
- Hamstrings

This is a classic runner's stretch with a literal twist. With the addition of a side bend, the move becomes multifaceted and much more efficient.

HOW TO DO IT: Sit down on the floor with one leg outstretched in front of you, the other bent with the foot resting on the inner thigh of the outstretched leg. Sitting up straight and tall, rotate your upper body toward the bent leg, rest your opposite hand on the thigh of the bent leg, then reach the other hand overhead and bend to the side. You should feel a good stretch in your side. Hold for thirty seconds to two minutes. Switch sides.

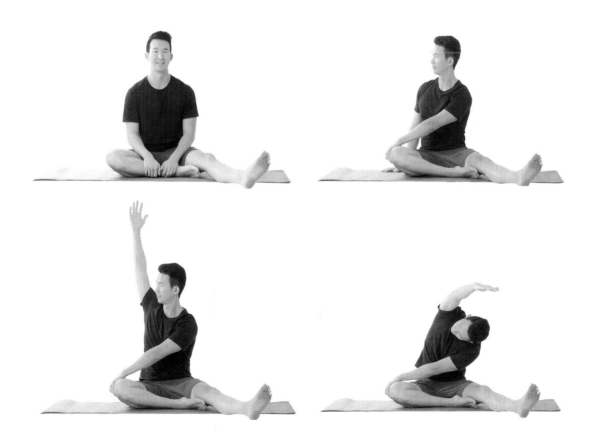

WALL HIP TAPS

Most of us favor one side of the body. This stretch helps equalize both sides. The farther away from the wall you stand while doing it, the deeper your stretch will be.

CUES

- Keep your back flat.
- Allow your opposite hand to slide down your leg as you stretch.

TARGET AREAS

- Low back
- Lats
- Obliques

 HOW TO DO IT: Stand straight and tall, with your side next to a wall. Take one small step away from the wall, raise your inside arm overhead, and tap your hip to the wall. Do ten reps. Switch sides.

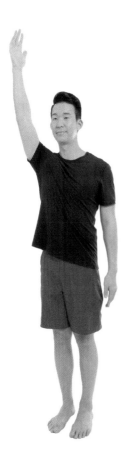 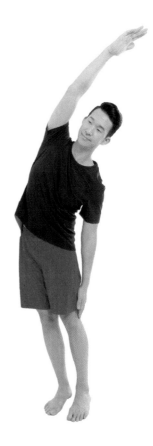

SKATER STRETCH

Named for the way your back leg glides behind you just like Wayne Gretzky's or Michelle Kwan's on the ice, this move stretches virtually the entire side of your body.

CUE

- Your front knee bends to enable the stretch.

TARGET AREAS

- Low back
- Lats
- Obliques

HOW TO DO IT: Stand straight and tall, with your side about one foot away from a wall. Place your inside palm on the wall, and slide your inside leg across and behind you as if curtsying. Hold for thirty seconds to two minutes. Switch sides.

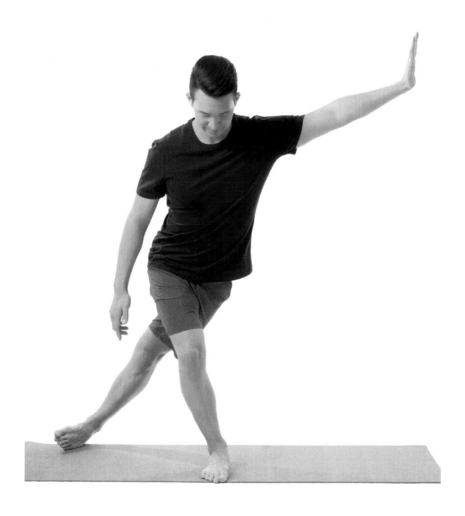

— 6

STRETCHES FOR THE MID- AND UPPER BACK

Your mid- and upper back extends from the middle of your spine to your neck—and seems to take a lot of the brunt of gravity. Maybe it's because we carry the weight of the world (or whatever life issues we come up against) on our shoulders, which then adds tension to the back. Add in the fact that many people hunch, whether over a desk at work or a steering wheel while driving, or just as part of their posture, and it's no wonder that so many of us feel tight and inflexible in the midback and develop knots between the shoulder blades.

The mid- and upper back is made up of the thoracic spine (also known as the *T-spine*), the latissimus dorsi (lats), the rhomboids, and the trapezii (plural for more than one *trapezius*; also called *traps*). The job of the T-spine is to help the body flex forward, extend backward, and rotate from side to side. If it's stiff and you cannot do either properly, you may feel the strain in your neck and lower back.

The trapezii, which are located in the middle of the upper back and attach to the neck, are tasked with moving the shoulders, head, and neck. That's a lot of responsibility, and they can easily get overworked. If you hold anything (like a baby or a bag of groceries) for a long time, repeatedly lift anything heavy (like boxes or a barbell), or manifest stress by holding your shoulders up by your ears in a perpetual shrug, the traps are going to get stiff and inflexible. (I'll also address the traps in chapter 9, which is devoted to the neck.)

Stretches that elongate the T-spine area not only keep the mid- and upper back muscles limber, they tend to feel especially relaxing. Something about the way you extend and flex the back in the T-Spine Cat/Cow Stretch seems to help tension melt away.

T-Spine

The T-spine, or thoracic spine, is the part of the spine that runs between the neck and the lower back and is the only part of the spine that connects to the rib cage. Most of us don't even notice when the T-spine is tight, but if you're ever asked to do a slight backbend in a yoga class or even just want to lean back to watch a beautiful bird fly overhead, you may suddenly become aware that your movement is limited.

But even if you don't take yoga or go in much for birdwatching, the T-spine needs to be able to flex and extend, side bend a little, and rotate to facilitate your daily movements. If it's stiff, all the muscles around it need to work extra hard to take up the slack. Inevitably, that puts excess pressure on the lower back and sometimes the neck—and they'll get the blame for your discomfort, even when the real culprit is the T-spine. So let's help it loosen it up.

WHAT ARE YOU IMPROVING?
Flexibility of the mid- and upper back.

ADDED BENEFIT
Taking pressure off the neck and lower back muscles.

CAT/COW STRETCH

This stretch is about the back, but you also get great movement in your hips. As you go into cat position (so named, as you probably figured out, because it looks like a cat rounding its back), your head leads the way by pulling in toward your chest. For the cow position (it looks like a cow's slightly sunken back), your low back arches, your head lifts, and your shoulders follow.

 HOW TO DO IT: Get down on all fours, knees under your hips, wrists under your shoulders. Tuck your chin and round your upper back; hold for two seconds. From there, look up, draw your shoulders back and drop your chest toward the floor, slightly arching your back; hold for two seconds. Do ten reps.

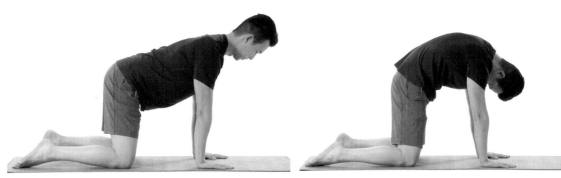

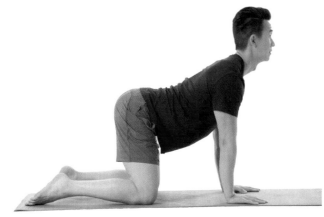

T-SPINE CAT/COW STRETCH

This variation on the Cat/Cow Stretch is a little more focused on the upper back than the traditional exercise. Both provide a great way to warm up before exercise.

CUES

- Sitting back on your heels takes the lower back out of the equation.
- Lead with your head, but don't overbend or arch your neck.
- Place pillow between butt and heels to take pressure off the knees.

TARGET AREA

- T-spine

HOW TO DO IT: Sit back on your heels, toes touching, knees slightly apart. Place your arms out in front of you at a 45-degree angle to your body, hands flat on the floor. Tuck your chin and round your upper back; hold for two seconds. From there, look up toward the ceiling, draw your shoulders back, and bring your chest toward the floor, neutralizing your upper spine; hold for two seconds. Do ten reps.

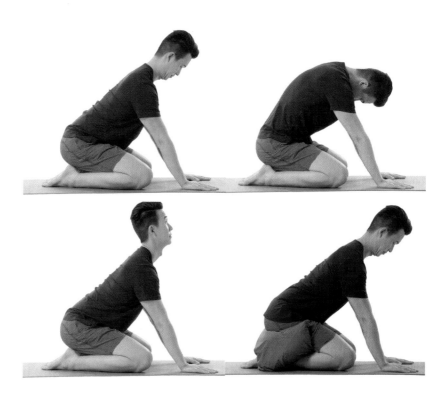

CAT/COW STRETCH
(Standing)

Unlike the Cat/Cow Stretch that's done while on your knees, this variation can be done almost anywhere. It's also a good alternative if you have tender knees.

CUES

- Keep your hands in front of you.
- Slowly ease into the movements.

TARGET AREA

- T-spine

HOW TO DO IT: From a standing position, push your hips back, bend your knees slightly, and place your palms on your thighs just above the knee. Tuck your chin and round your upper back. Hold for two seconds. From there, look up, push your chest forward, and draw your shoulders back, slightly arching your back; hold for two seconds. Do ten reps.

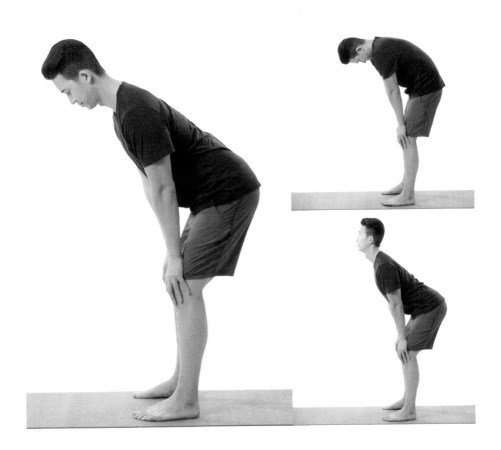

CAT/COW STRETCH
(Seated)

CUE
- Slowly ease into the movements.

TARGET AREA
- T-spine

Yet another variation on the Cat/Cow theme, you can do this one seated in a chair or cross-legged on the floor. Why so many Cat/Cows? Depending on your body, one of them may feel better to you than the others or (in the case of the Standing Cat/Cow Stretch) simply be more convenient. Try them all, then stick with the one you most enjoy.

HOW TO DO IT: Sit on the floor with your legs crossed and your hands resting on your shins. Look up, push your chest forward, clasp your hands in front of you, and draw your shoulders back, slightly arching your back; hold for two seconds. From there, tuck your chin and round your upper back. Hold for two seconds. Do ten reps.

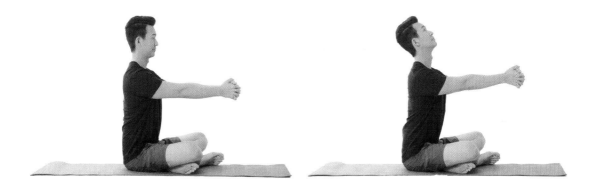

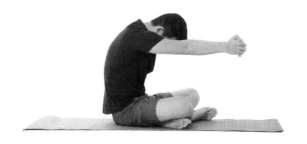

T-SPINE ROTATION
(On All Fours)

Every time you twist around—to grab something, to see who's calling your name—you're rotating your spine. Again, as I have mentioned in regard to other body parts, we need to be able to move smoothly in all directions. By getting the T-spine to rotate, this exercise has you covered.

 HOW TO DO IT: Get down on all fours, knees under your hips, wrists under your shoulders. Place one hand behind your head, elbow out to the side. In one smooth move, rotate your upper body down to bring your elbow toward the floor, then push your opposite hand into the floor and rotate the other way to bring your elbow up toward the ceiling. Do ten reps. Switch sides.

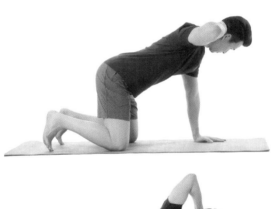

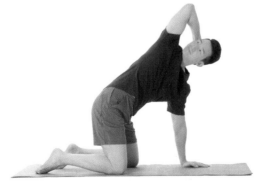

T-SPINE ROTATION
(Sitting on Heels)

T-Spine Rotation (On All Fours) is great, but maybe you want to isolate the T-spine even more. Sit your butt onto your heels! Sitting makes it tougher to rotate from the low back, allowing you to really target the mid-upper back. If it's difficult to sit back on your heels, place a rolled-up towel or foam roller between your butt and heels.

CUES
- Your back is in a neutral position.
- Keep your lower body as still as possible as you rotate.

TARGET AREA
- T-spine

HOW TO DO IT: Sit back on your heels, toes touching, knees slightly apart. Place one hand on the floor in front of you, arm locked, and the other hand behind your head, elbow out to the side. In one smooth move, rotate your upper body down to bring your elbow toward the floor, then push your hand into the floor, and rotate the opposite way to bring your elbow up toward the ceiling. Do ten reps. Switch sides.

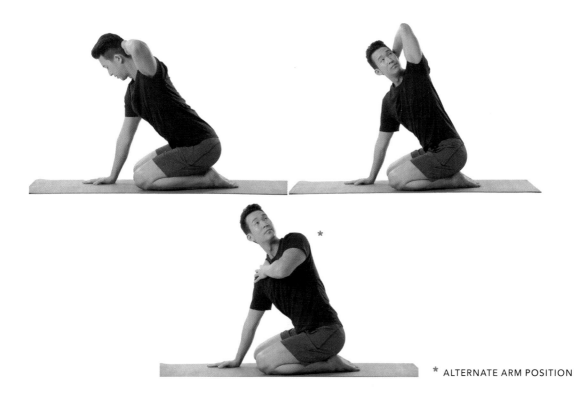

* ALTERNATE ARM POSITION

T-SPINE EXTENSION ON WALL (Standing)

This very simple stretch works wonders on a back that's been pressed up against a chair all day.

CUES

- Bending the knees takes the hamstrings out of play.
- Your head stays in a neutral position.

TARGET AREAS

- T-spine
- Lats

HOW TO DO IT: Stand about six inches farther than arm's length in front of a wall. Bend your knees slightly, and lean forward to place your hands on the wall. Push your hips back, and drop your chest toward the floor until you feel a good stretch in your back. Hold for thirty seconds to two minutes or perform 10 reps.

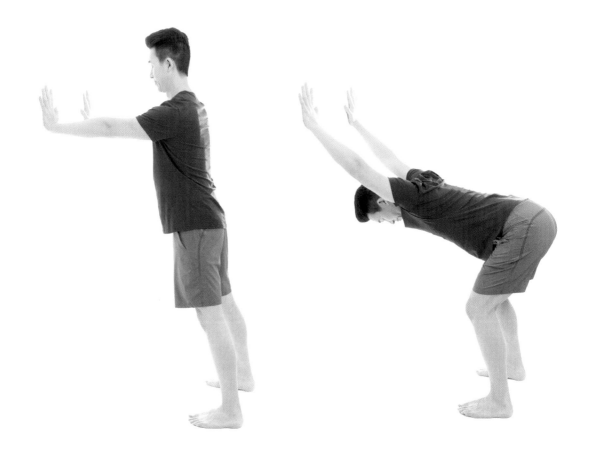

T-SPINE EXTENSION ON WALL (Tall-Kneeling)

You should never feel bad about how far you can—or can't—go in a stretch. We all have different bodies; the goal is to maximize the flexibility you do have. Still, some stretches can feel like you're hitting a wall, which is why I love this one; it just feels effortless. See if you agree.

CUE

- Your head stays in a neutral position.

TARGET AREAS

- T-spine
- Lats

 HOW TO DO IT: Kneel about six inches farther than arm's length in front of a wall, toes tucked under. Lean forward, place your hands on the wall, then push your hips back over your legs and drop your chest toward the floor until you feel a good stretch in the back. Hold for thirty seconds to two minutes or perform 10 reps.

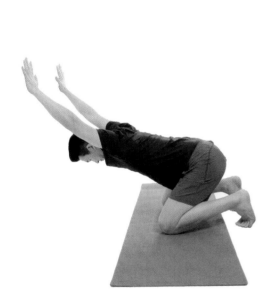 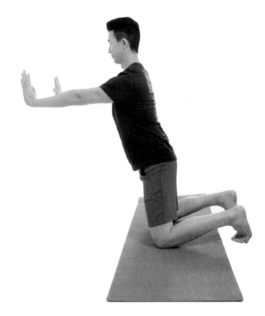

PUPPY POSE

You've heard of downward dog, the classic yoga pose? This is kind of a mini version that gets deep into the midback.

CUE

- The farther forward your hands, the greater the stretch.

TARGET AREAS

- T-spine
- Lats
- Abs

 HOW TO DO IT: Get down on all fours, knees under your hips, wrists under your shoulders. Walk your hands forward, and drop your chest until you feel a good stretch in your midback. Hold for thirty seconds to two minutes.

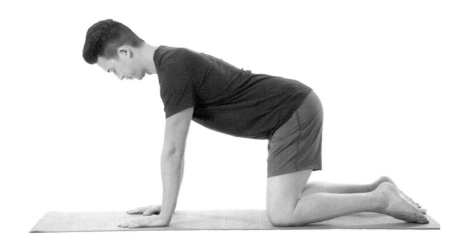

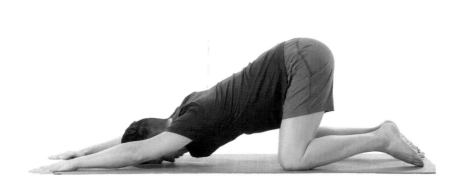

T-SPINE WINDMILL STRETCH (Half-Kneeling)

This dynamic stretch uses a wall for guidance, but it's not absolutely necessary. If you don't have a bare wall to position yourself next to, just perform the exercise without it, taking care to keep your arm in the same plane as it windmills.

CUES

- To make the movement easier, move farther away from the wall.
- Your upper body stays tall.

TARGET AREAS

- T-spine
- Shoulders

HOW TO DO IT: Kneel next to a wall with your outside leg bent at a 90-degree angle, foot flat on the floor. Raise your arms in front of you, with your inside arm on the wall. Rotate your upper body toward the wall to bring the arm on the wall up and over in an arc (as you hit the midpoint, your palm will turn to face the wall). Reverse the motion and come back to starting position. Do ten reps. Switch sides.

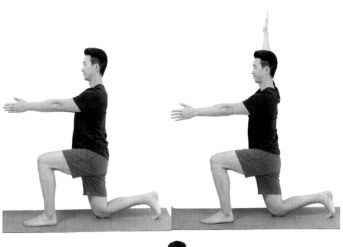

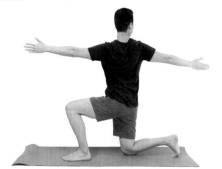

T-SPINE WINDMILL STRETCH (Side-Lying)

At first glance, this dynamic stretch might seem the same as the T-Spine Windmill Stretch (Half-Kneeling), but the arm movements are actually different. You can choose to do one or the other, but if you have particularly tight shoulders, consider doing both to take your shoulder joint through a fuller range of motion.

- Place a pillow under your head for support if needed.

- T-spine
- Pecs
- Shoulders

HOW TO DO IT: Lie on the floor on your side with your knees drawn up to hip level. Place your bottom hand just above your knees to pin them to the floor. Take your top arm across your body at shoulder level, then rotate your upper body to bring the arm to the other side (still at shoulder level). Reverse the motion and come back to starting position. Do ten reps. Switch sides.

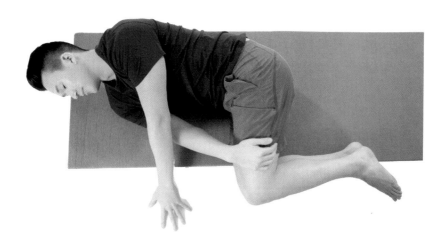

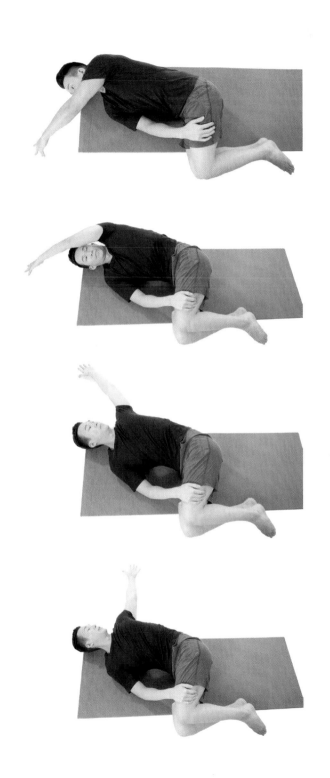

T-SPINE EXTENSION ON A BENCH

CUE

- Keep your elbows in line with your shoulders.

TARGET AREAS

- T-spine
- Lats
- Triceps

One of the few exercises in this book that calls for a prop, this T-Spine Extension can also be done without the stick. If you do have something handy (even the tube inside a wrapping paper roll will do), I recommend using it to help keep your hands the same distance apart during the stretch.

HOW TO DO IT: Kneel about a foot and a half away from a bench or low table. Holding a stick between your hands shoulder-width apart, place your elbows on the seat of the bench. Shift your hips back over your legs, and bring the stick behind your back as you sink your chest toward the floor. Do 10 reps.

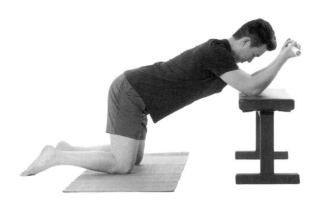

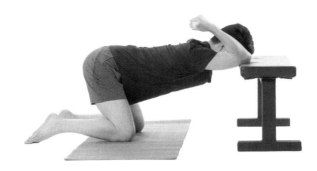

OPEN BOOK

By rotating the spine, this stretch is designed to get you out of your two-direction comfort zone.

 HOW TO DO IT: Supporting your head with a pillow or mat, lie on your side with both knees drawn up at a 90-degree angle at hip level. Extend both arms at chest level, hands together, and elbows locked. Keeping your bottom arm on the floor, swing your top arm up and over to the floor on the other side of your body. Hold for thirty seconds to two minutes.

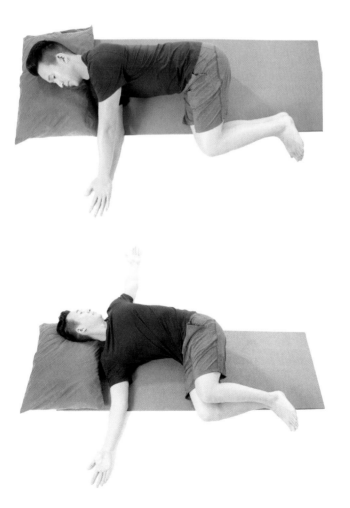

Lats

Can you easily raise your arms overhead? If not, then your lats (latissimus dorsi) are likely to blame. The lats, located midback, are big and wrap around the side of the body. They help you move your shoulders and do things like pull a door open. But when they're tight, they can pull your shoulders forward and hinder a whole lot of different movements. Trying to get your bag into the carry-on compartment on a plane. Swimming. Using the lat pull-down machine at the gym. If it's difficult to get your arms overhead, you're probably going to arch your back to make it happen, and that can end up causing pain.

WHAT ARE YOU IMPROVING?
Flexibility in the side back muscles.

ADDED BENEFIT
Improves posture.

CHILD'S POSE WITH SIDE BEND

Just by moving your arms to the side, you can turn the by-now-familiar Child's Pose into a stretch for the muscles that run down the side of your back.

CUES

- Widen your legs as much as you'd like; this is a personal choice.
- As you loosen up, shimmy your hands forward for a more intense stretch.

TARGET AREAS

- Back
- Lats

HOW TO DO IT: Sit back on your heels, toes touching, knees apart. Lower your upper body over your knees, stretch your arms forward, and place your forehead on the floor. Shimmy both arms to one side until you feel a good stretch in your midback. Hold for thirty seconds to two minutes. Switch sides.

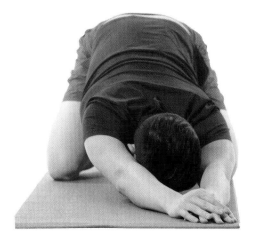
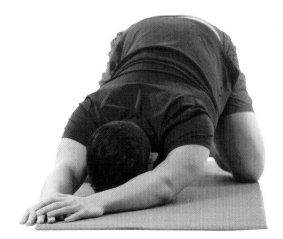

SIDE BEND STRETCH
(Standing)

When you do this basic stretch, resist the urge to rotate; keep your upper body straight.

CUE

- Shift hips to one side while reaching your arms toward each other.

TARGET AREA

- Lats

 HOW TO DO IT: Stand straight and tall, feet shoulder-width apart. Raise your arms, place your fingertips together, and bend to one side until you feel a good stretch on the opposite side. Hold for thirty seconds to two minutes. Switch sides.

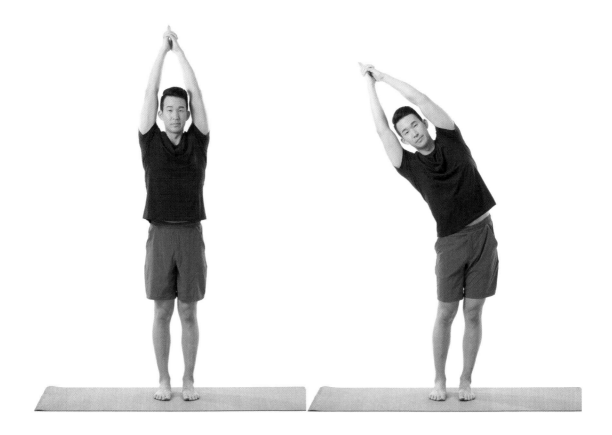

Rhomboids

The rhomboids start at the spine and go into your shoulder blade. They help keep your shoulders back; the healthier your rhomboids, the better your posture. Avid computer users and other people who sit at desks for a long time are prone to rounding their shoulders forward, which in turn overstretches the rhomboids. So why am I including rhomboid stretches? For one thing, not everyone has rounded shoulders, so you may not even have the overstretching problem. For another, as you do the stretches and strengtheners in this book and improve your overall flexibility, you'll be less likely to round your shoulders at your desk. That means your rhomboids will be normal (or even tight) and in need of maintenance stretching. Plus, these rhomboid stretches feel really good.

WHAT ARE YOU IMPROVING?
Flexibility in the muscles that pull the shoulder blades together.

ADDED BENEFIT
Improves posture.

THREADING THE NEEDLE

There are not too many ways to stretch the rhomboids, but you don't need a quantity of exercises—just a few quality ones like Threading the Needle. It does the trick.

CUE

- Play with your supporting arm to find the position that feels best.

TARGET AREAS

- Back
- Shoulders
- T-spine

 HOW TO DO IT: Get down on all fours, knees under your hips, wrists under your shoulders. Slide one arm under your body and stretch it to the other side. Bend the supporting arm or slide it slightly forward to steady your weight. You should feel a good stretch in your shoulder blade. Hold for thirty seconds to two minutes. Switch sides.

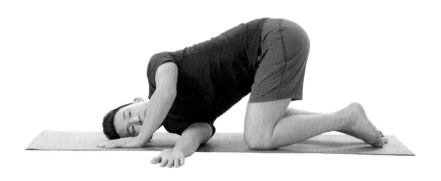

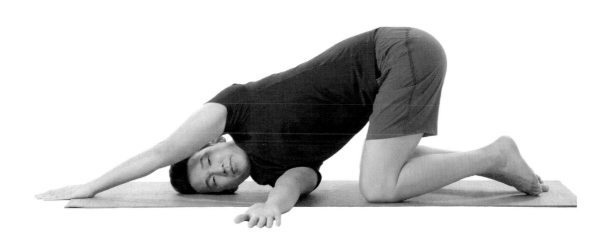

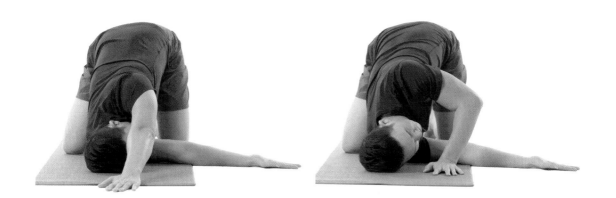

CROSS-BODY STRETCH

I prefer to do this stretch while standing, but you can also do it while sitting.

CUE

- Try not to rotate your upper body.

TARGET AREAS

- Back
- Shoulders

 HOW TO DO IT: Stand straight and tall, feet shoulder-width apart. Swing one arm across your body at chest level, and lightly push into it with your opposite hand until you feel a good stretch in the back of the arm. Hold for thirty seconds to two minutes. Switch sides.

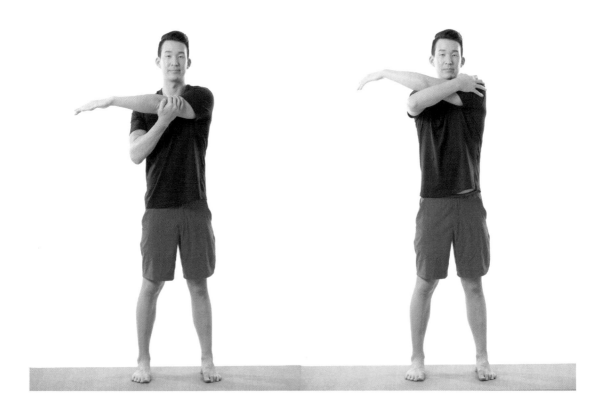

— 7

STRETCHES FOR THE SHOULDERS AND CHEST

We pay a lot more attention to the fronts of our bodies than our backsides. This is particularly true when we exercise, with some of us working the "mirror muscles" more than their counterparts on the other side of the body. This imbalance of attention can lead to a rolling forward of the shoulders, tight pectoral muscles (pecs), and eventual discomfort.

The shoulders in particular can be a trouble spot. They seem to be related to our state of mind. If we're stressed and tense, they're up around our ears. If we're sad, they droop. If we're worried, they cave forward. It's a lot of stress to put on one body part! The exercises in this chapter not only help stretch and so ease these muscles, they also work on mobility. The muscles surrounding the scapulae—your shoulder blades—need a good range of motion if you hope to be able to move your arms as needed. The same goes for the rotator cuff, a group of muscles and tendons that surround the shoulder joint.

The other muscles you're going to stretch in this section are the pecs, or pectoralis major and pectoralis minor, which are spread over the breastbone. These muscles contribute to the rounding forward that occurs with too much desk sitting. Tending to them will help you keep your shoulders back and perhaps, because they are the muscles that expand when you inhale, even help you breathe easier.

Shoulders and Chest

The shoulder joints—like the hips—don't move in only one plane. They need to be able to move in all directions so you can do things like reach the top shelf to put groceries away, turn and grab something off a table behind you, and throw a ball with your kid in the yard. Besides elongating the muscles in the shoulders and chest, the stretches in this section will also help you improve mobility in this area of the body. You know those people who approach the world with their shoulders back (not rigid like a drill sergeant's but in a confident way) and an easiness in their bodies? You'll be one of them.

WHAT ARE YOU IMPROVING?
Mobility in the shoulder muscles and flexibility in the chest.

ADDED BENEFITS
Provides relief of shoulder pain; improves posture.

WALL ANGELS

If you tend to feel like you're hunched over all the time, make this your go-to movement for combatting bad posture. It's awesome for your back and shoulders and also opens up your chest. Make sure to keep your body on the wall throughout the movement. If it's a struggle, try Floor Angels (next page).

(next page)

CUE

- Engage your abs to flatten your lower back to the wall.

TARGET AREAS

- Shoulders
- Pecs

HOW TO DO IT: Stand straight and tall, with your back against a wall, your lower back as flat as possible, and the back of your head touching the wall. Bring your elbows to the wall and out to the side at shoulder level, bent at a 90-degree angle, with your forearms flat on the wall. Straighten your arms, and slide them up the wall. Hold for two to five seconds, then slide them back to starting position. Do ten reps.

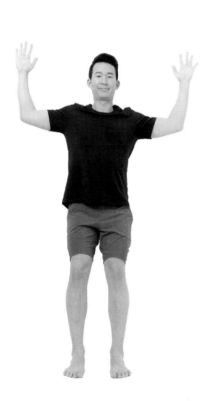
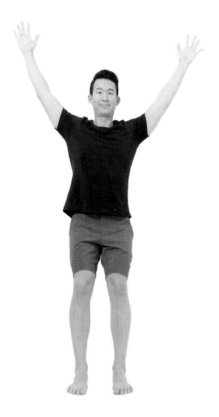

FLOOR ANGELS

This is a variation of Wall Angels, which is itself a variation of snow play. Doing the move on the floor provides some extra support without diminishing the stretch's effectiveness in the least.

CUE

- Engage your abs to flatten your lower back to the floor.

TARGET AREAS

- Shoulders
- Pecs

HOW TO DO IT: Lie on the floor faceup with your lower back as flat as possible, knees bent, feet flat on the floor. Bring your elbows to the floor and out to the side at shoulder level, bent at a 90-degree angle, with your forearms flat on the floor. Straighten your arms, and slide them overhead. Hold for two to five seconds, then slide them back to starting position. Do ten reps.

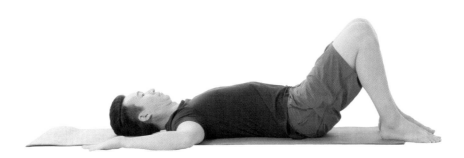

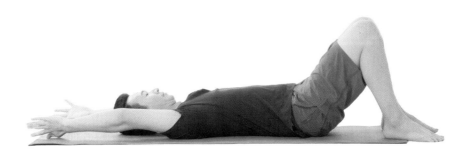

PROTRACTION AND RETRACTION STRETCH

It's important to keep the muscles attached to the shoulder blades (scapulae) strong so the shoulders stay injury-free. But our shoulders also need to be able to move freely and easily. That's where protraction and retraction come in. Retraction refers to pulling the shoulder blade back (imagine squeezing your shoulder blades onto your back); protraction refers to reaching the shoulder blade forward. By exaggerating moves you make naturally, this stretch ensures that there's no tightness in the area as you go about your daily business of living.

CUE

- The forward-and-back move is subtle.

TARGET AREAS

- Trapezii
- Rhomboids
- Serratus anterior

HOW TO DO IT: Stand about a foot from a wall, then lean forward and place your palms flat on the wall so you are in a push-up position. Keeping your hands on the wall, pull your shoulder blades back and hold for two to five seconds. Push them forward into starting position. Do ten reps.

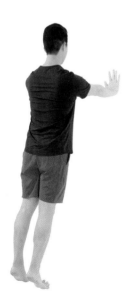
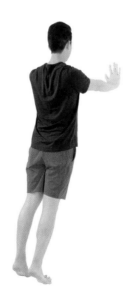
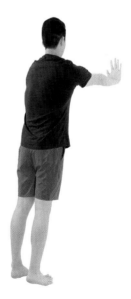

PEC STRETCH ON WALL

If your shoulders roll forward, the first thing you might think about doing is rolling your shoulders back. Good idea. Now here is another one: Work on opening up the pectoral muscles in your chest. One of the pec muscles attaches to the top of the shoulder blade, and when it is tight, it can pull the shoulders forward. You might not even think your chest muscles are tight, but once you get into this stretch, you'll likely notice it in a big way. It gets in there deep.

CUE

- Lean into the doorway or wall slightly to deepen the stretch.

TARGET AREAS

- Pecs
- Shoulders

HOW TO DO IT: Stand with one arm bent at a 90-degree angle at shoulder height against the frame of a doorway or wall. Rotate your upper body slightly until you feel a good stretch in your chest. Hold for thirty seconds to two minutes. Switch sides.

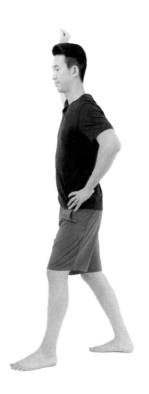
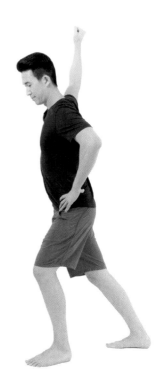

DYNAMIC PEC STRETCH
(Half-Kneeling)

This book, as you have no doubt noticed, features a lot of stretches done while kneeling, either on one leg or two. I sometimes provide a direction about how to position the foot (or feet) of your kneeling leg(s), and other times, I do not. This is one of those instances in which I do not provide direction, and the reason is because it doesn't influence the stretch. You can flex your toes so your heel is up or lay the front of your foot on the floor. Play around with it and see which way feels most comfortable.

CUE

- The farther you lean in, the deeper the stretch.

TARGET AREAS

- Pecs
- Shoulders

HOW TO DO IT: Kneel on one leg next to a wall, outer leg bent at a 90-degree angle, and foot flat on the floor. Bend your inside arm at a 90-degree angle, and place your forearm and side of your hand on the wall. Slide your upper body forward slightly until you feel a good stretch in your chest. Hold for thirty seconds to two minutes. Switch sides.

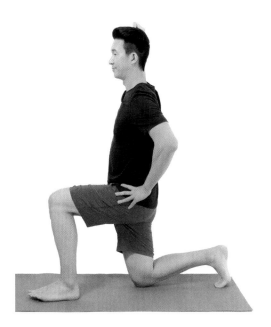

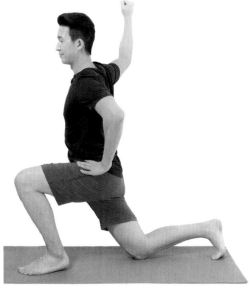

SCORPION STRETCH

This is called the Scorpion Stretch because the body position is reminiscent of the little arachnid (yes, scorpions are related to spiders). Is it also deadly? Hardly, but it does pack a good punch in the chest- and shoulder-stretching area!

 HOW TO DO IT: Lie facedown on the floor with your arms at shoulder height or slightly higher. Lift one leg up and cross it over the other leg until your toes hit the floor and you feel a good stretch in your chest. (The arm on the side of the leg you cross over will naturally bend as you rotate.)

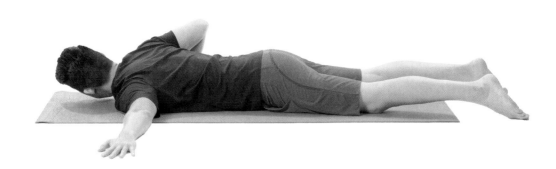

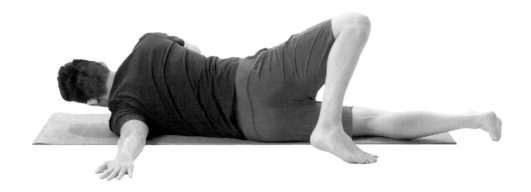

WALL SLIDE WITH SHOULDER LIFT-OFF

This is a great active movement that will help you increase shoulder mobility as well as improve your posture. Using a wall to do this exercise helps you maintain good form.

CUES

- Your feet can stay together, or you can place one foot back.
- Don't allow your back to arch.
- Your head stays level.

TARGET AREAS

- Biceps
- Shoulders

HOW TO DO IT: Stand facing a wall, and place your forearms on the wall, palms facing each other and elbows at shoulder height. Maintaining a straight back, slide your forearms up the wall. As your forearms and hands come off the wall, pull your arms back so they are above your shoulders. Bring your hands back to the wall, and slowly slide your forearms back to the starting position. Do ten reps.

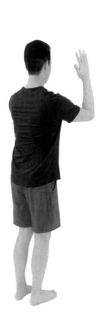
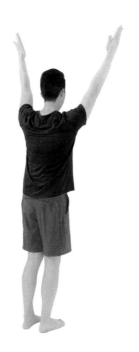
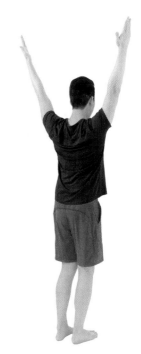

— 8

STRETCHES FOR THE ARMS

When I talk about the arms, I'm also talking about the hands, even though these usually get left out of any talk about flexibility. Most people use their hands continuously, especially if their work entails a lot of typing or something like cutting hair or construction. In this chapter, I address all the parts of the arm: the biceps (front of the upper arm), triceps (the back of the upper arm), the forearms, and the hands. These stretches will be especially important for you if you have issues like tennis or golf elbow, or nerve-related pain like carpal tunnel and other types of wrist tenderness.

Biceps

Besides being the universal symbol of strength, the biceps, when contracted, play a critical role in helping you lift anything—a dumbbell, a laundry basket, the box you ordered from Amazon, a coffee cup. Anything and just about everything. Here you're going to pay some attention to extending rather than contracting them. This will keep them loose and ready to take on any of the million tasks a day you ask of them.

WHAT ARE YOU IMPROVING?
Flexibility in the front upper arm muscles.

ADDED BENEFIT
Provides greater length in the arms when reaching.

BICEPS STRETCH
(Kneeling)

Biceps get a lot of love when it comes to strengthening, but not so much when it comes to stretching. This exercise targets the muscles, while also giving the chest and shoulders good elongation.

CUES

- Knees stay under your hips.
- Arms are straight to your sides.

TARGET AREAS

- Biceps
- Pecs
- Shoulders

 HOW TO DO IT: Get down on your hands and knees and place your hands on the floor about twice shoulder-width apart to support your upper body. Bend one elbow, and, keeping the other arm straight, rotate your upper body and bring the shoulder of the straight arm down toward the floor until you feel a good stretch in the front of your arm and chest. Hold for thirty seconds to two minutes. Switch sides.

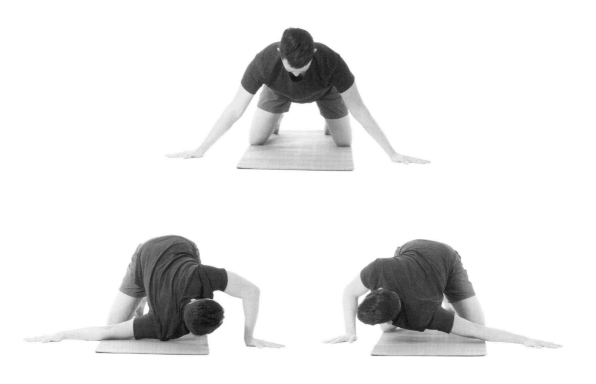

BICEPS STRETCH ON WALL

It's difficult to isolate the biceps, but that just means your stretch can be multifaceted. This stretch also engages the pec muscles, making it another two-for-the-price-of-one move.

CUE

- Your upper body stays straight and tall.

TARGET AREAS

- Biceps
- Pecs

 HOW TO DO IT: Stand with your side about a foot from a wall. Place your inside hand flat on the wall at shoulder height, then rotate your torso away from the wall until you feel a good stretch in your chest and arm. Hold for thirty seconds to two minutes. Switch sides.

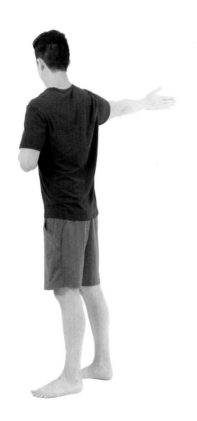 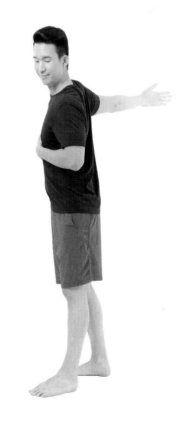

Triceps

Your triceps, the muscles in the back of your upper arm, and your elbow are intimately acquainted. The triceps allow you to extend your elbow. The biceps pull it in; the triceps bring it back down. The triceps is one of those muscles that you probably won't know is tight until you stretch it. Once you're in a triceps stretch, you'll likely see how much you need it.

WHAT ARE YOU IMPROVING?
Flexibility in the back upper arm muscles.

ADDED BENEFITS
Provides greater length in the arms when reaching; facilitates easier shoulder movement.

TRICEPS STRETCH
(Standing)

This is another one of those anytime-anywhere stretches. It's a great exercise to add to your regimen (especially if you engage in arm-centric sports like squash, tennis, rowing, or swimming), but it's also one that you can just sneak in while you're, say, standing in line or watching TV.

CUE

- Push your elbow down gently.

TARGET AREAS

- Triceps
- Lats

HOW TO DO IT: Standing straight and tall, raise one arm, bend it at the elbow, and drop your hand behind the middle of your back. Take your other hand and grab the raised elbow and gently push it down until you feel a good stretch in the back of your arm. Hold for thirty seconds to two minutes. Switch sides.

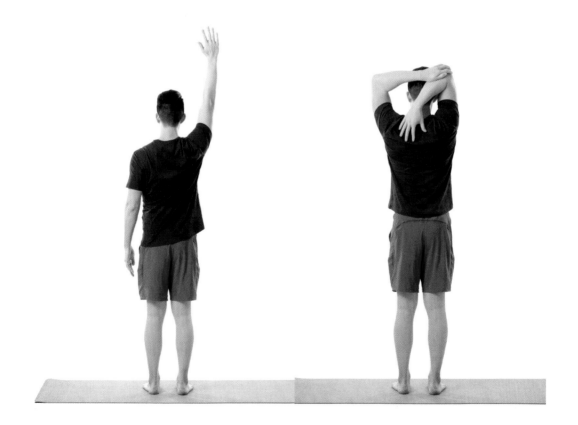

CHILD'S POSE WITH TRICEPS

Another variation on Child's Pose, this one allows you to extend the back-of-the-arm muscles while sinking into a relaxing position.

CUE

- Pressing your elbows down into the floor will deepen the stretch.

TARGET AREAS

- Triceps
- Back
- Lats

HOW TO DO IT: Sit back on your heels, toes touching, knees apart. Lower your upper body between your knees, stretch your arms forward, and place your forehead on or near the floor. Bend your elbows, and bring your hands to your back just below your neck. You should feel a good stretch in the back of your arms. Hold for thirty seconds to two minutes.

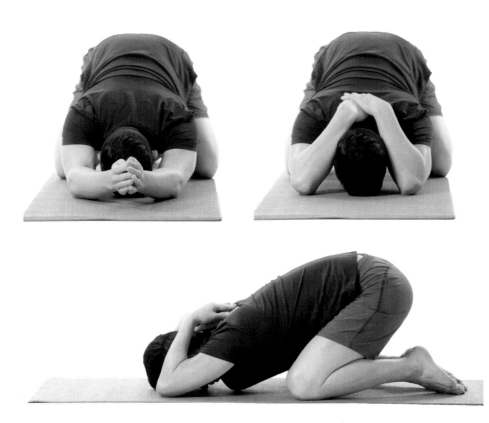

Forearms and Hands

In this world, biceps get the bright lights (thank you, Arnold Schwarzenegger), while the forearms and hands go unsung. Yet if you work at a computer, think about how much you use them. If you have a job in which you're always grabbing things or if you work out with dumbbells at a gym, your forearms and hands are getting taxed. Here, as with so many other muscles in the body, tightness can be the end result. You may even begin experiencing pain in your wrists and elbows. These stretches can help ease and prevent the pain and are like applying a soothing gel to smaller but still workhorse muscles.

WHAT ARE YOU IMPROVING?
Flexibility in the lower arm muscles and hands.

ADDED BENEFITS
Lessens the risk of carpal tunnel and elbow issues.

FOREARM STRETCH
(Kneeling) (Flexors)

This exercise gets you to do something you probably normally don't: face your inner arms forward. By doing so, with hands flat on the floor, you get a remarkable stretch in this underserved area.

HOW TO DO IT: Kneel on the floor. Extend your arms in front of you, rotate them, and extend your hands at the wrist so the insides of your forearms are facing up and your fingertips are facing down. Keeping your arms in this position, move to all fours. Your palms should now be flat on the floor with fingers facing toward you, and you should feel a good stretch in your inner forearms. Hold for thirty seconds to two minutes.

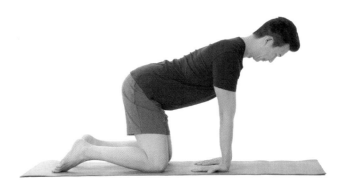

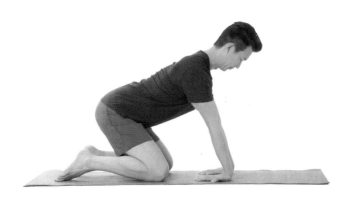

FOREARM STRETCH
(Kneeling) (Extensors)

The Forearm Stretch (Kneeling) (Flexors) and
this exercise are like two sides of the same coin.
Together, they limber up both sides of the forearm.

CUE

- Shift your hips back over your
  heels to deepen the stretch.

TARGET AREAS

- Forearms
- Wrists

HOW TO DO IT: Kneel on the floor. Extend your arms in front of you, then flex your hands at the wrists so your fingers are pointing back. Keeping your arms in this position, move to all fours. The backs of your hands should now be flat on the floor, your fingers pointing toward you, and you should feel a good stretch in your outer forearms. Hold for thirty seconds to two minutes.

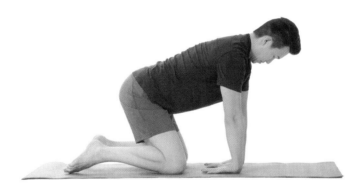

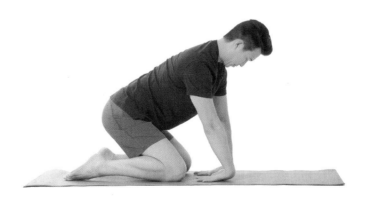

FINGER/HAND STRETCH

Take a break from your keyboard and do this stretch often. Will it make you a better typist? I can't promise that, but I believe your overworked hands will thank you.

CUE

- Use a gentle touch to pull your fingers.

TARGET AREAS

- Fingers
- Thumbs
- Hands
- Wrists

 HOW TO DO IT: While sitting or standing, outstretch one arm in front of you at shoulder height. Extend your hand at the wrist, fingers pointing up, then place the palm of your other hand on your four fingers and gently pull them back. Hold for thirty seconds to two minutes. Repeat with your thumb. Switch sides.

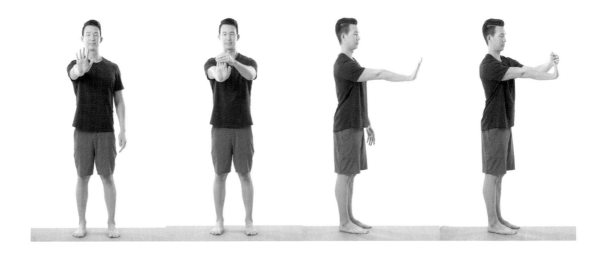

CARPAL TUNNEL RELIEF

There is a small tunnel from the wrist to the hand that allows a nerve, called the median nerve, to pass from the arm to the fingers. When the nerve gets compressed or irritated, it can cause pain, tingling, or numbness—carpal tunnel syndrome. If you type a lot without using proper ergonomics—that is, your wrists are bent for long periods of time—or you do any other type of repetitive wrist movements, you are a candidate for carpal tunnel syndrome.

The hand stretches in this chapter will help make it less likely that you'll experience the symptoms of carpal tunnel syndrome. This particular stretch can also ease discomfort in the thumb and the two fingers next to it (top part of hand, palm side). It helps the median nerve glide through the tunnel and the other structures it passes.

CARPAL TUNNEL NERVE GLIDE

Besides helping take the pressure off the nerve, this exercise gives your neck a nice stretch, too.

CUE

- If a deep bend at the wrist is painful, back off and do as much as you can.

HOW TO DO IT: While sitting or standing, extend one arm out to the side at shoulder level, palm facing up. Bend your wrist so your fingers face down, and at the same time, tilt your head to the same side. Hold for a second. Reverse the motion and bend your wrist so your fingers point up, and at the same time, tilt your head to the other side. Perform ten to fifteen reps.

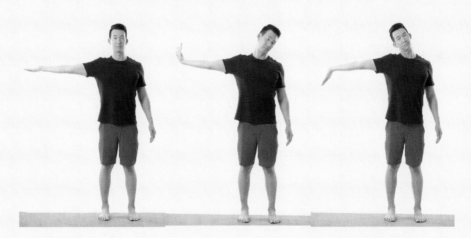

— 9

STRETCHES FOR THE NECK

Think about those muscles holding up your head, all day, every day. They deserve some love for all that hard work! These muscles, which include the trapezius (see chapter 6) and several others with awesome names (sternocleidomastoid! splenius cervicis!—don't worry, there's no reason for you to remember them), seem to get kinked up like no others. I see a lot of clients who have stiff necks—they can be caused by so many things, including sleeping with your head in an awkward position or just day-to-day stress—but stretching to improve range of motion helps clear things up pretty quickly. The exercises in this chapter are very soothing.

Neck

Neck stretches are not necessarily what you'd expect them to be. That's because to properly stretch the neck, you don't just stretch the neck; you also stretch the surrounding muscles like the trapezii, which connect to the neck but run down the sides of the upper back. The exercises here also help you elongate the levator scapulae, which connects the scapula to the neck, and the sternocleidomastoid (SCM), which helps you rotate the head.

WHAT ARE YOU IMPROVING?
Mobility in the neck and surrounding muscles.

ADDED BENEFIT
Provides pain relief in the neck.

TRAP STRETCH

Sometimes subtle moves have a surprisingly big impact. Try doing this stretch without putting one arm behind your back (just keep it by your side), then try doing it as instructed. I think you'll feel a difference between the two, with the arm behind your back being the more potent stretch.

CUE

- Pull lightly; don't be too aggressive.

TARGET AREA

- Traps

HOW TO DO IT: While sitting or standing and keeping your upper body straight and tall, bend one arm at a 90-degree angle at the elbow, place it behind your back, and drop your shoulder down. Curl the other arm over your head, and with your hand at your ear, gently pull your head down toward your shoulder until you feel a good stretch down the side of your neck. Hold for thirty seconds to two minutes. Switch sides.

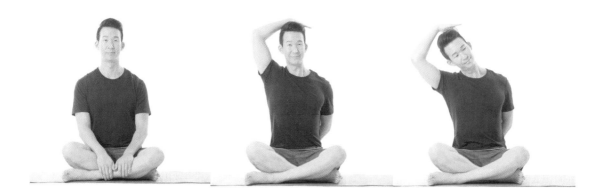

LEVATOR SCAPULAE STRETCH

The neck is relatively strong; after all, it holds your head up. Nonetheless, always take care when pulling or pushing your head into a stretch; go slowly and ease into it.

CUE

- Push lightly; don't be too aggressive.

TARGET AREAS

- Levator scapulae
- Traps
- Neck extensors

HOW TO DO IT: While sitting or standing and keeping your upper body straight and tall, bend one arm at a 90-degree angle at the elbow, place it behind your back, and drop your shoulder down. Place the oppposite hand on top of your head, turn your head to that side at about a 45-degree angle, and drop it down toward your chest. Gently push your head down with your hand until you feel a good stretch in the side/back of your neck. Hold for thirty seconds to two minutes. Switch sides.

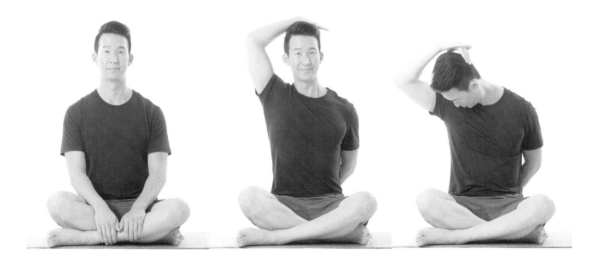

SCM STRETCH

As you drop your head back, close your eyes and luxuriate in the stretch for its duration. This one is a real tension reliever!

CUE

- Work slowly; there is no need to rush.

TARGET AREAS

- SCM
- Neck flexors
- Neck rotators

 HOW TO DO IT: While sitting or standing and keeping your upper body straight and tall, turn your head to one side and look over your shoulder. Slowly drop your head back until you feel a good stretch in the front of your neck. Hold for thirty seconds to two minutes. Switch sides.

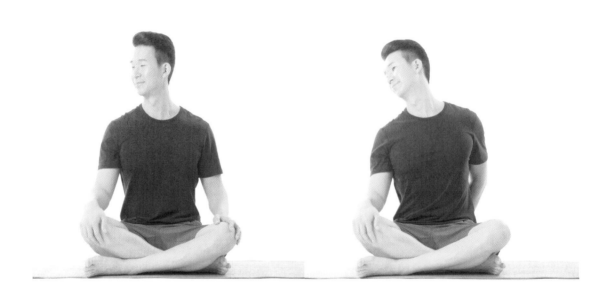

NECK EXTENSOR STRETCH

While how long you hold a stretch is your choice, I suggest trying to hold this one for the whole two minutes. Let it be a meditative time-out.

 HOW TO DO IT: While sitting or standing and keeping your upper body straight and tall, place one hand behind your head, and gently push your head down toward your chest. You should feel a good stretch in the back of your neck. Hold for thirty seconds to two minutes.

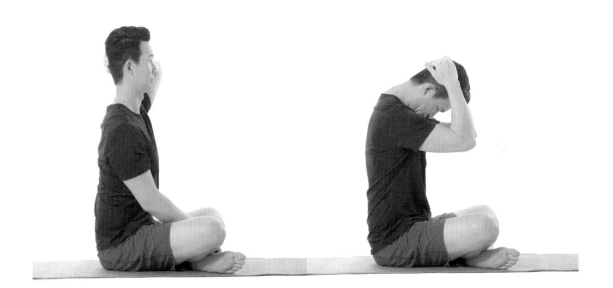

PART 2

STRENGTHENING, TOOLS, SPECIALTY ROUTINES

— 10 —

STRETCH-REINFORCING STRENGTHENERS

Recently, I looked up the word *brawn* in the dictionary: "physical strength in contrast to intelligence." No surprise there, I guess, since we all know the phrase "brains over brawn" and its variations. But in some ways, I also think the notion that the brain and physical strength are two completely different entities is wrong—and nothing proves the point better than the way that strength influences flexibility.

Let me backtrack a bit and reiterate why I have included an assortment of strengtheners in a book on stretching. One reason muscles get tight and inflexible is because they may be trying to protect themselves or the structures (like bones and joints) they surround or are attached to. So if the muscles in your back are weak and not quite up to the challenges they are facing because of your daily movements or a certain type of exercise you regularly engage in, they are going to get tense and inelastic. In a sense, they mimic what the whole body does when it's under threat. Even though it's somewhat of an exaggeration, if you think of the phrase *frozen in terror*, you get a sense of what I mean.

Now here is where the brain comes in. When you strengthen a muscle, it tells your brain that it's okay to use the flexibility it already has. Let's take someone who complains of tightness in the hamstrings. I will often ask a new client to lie on his back and raise one leg toward the ceiling as far as he can. I will then step in and support the leg and gently push it farther. If the leg can get close to perpendicular (it varies for everyone), then the tightness may be due to lack of strength. My client may have the ability to extend his hamstrings farther, but weakness is preventing the muscles from extending to their maximum. His brain is putting on the brakes, though my intervention clearly shows that the hamstrings are capable of stretching farther. If, however, those muscles are strong, the brain gets the message and sends it back to the hamstrings: you're good to go. Brawn and brain are connected after all.

Incorporating Strengtheners into a Stretch Routine

There are all kinds of ways to strengthen the body, weight training being the most effective way. Weight training (with either free weights or weight machines) builds and preserves muscle mass, the latter of which is especially important as we age and muscle tissue diminishes. Other forms of strength training, such as exercises that use bands or your own body weight for resistance, also build and preserve muscle mass, but not as well as weight training.

The strengtheners in this chapter rely on body weight for resistance, although you can certainly add weights to some of them (I'll tell you which ones as you go) right at the outset or as you get stronger. Why, if weight training is the most effective way to strengthen muscles, have I gone the body weight route? My goal is to provide you with exercises that will reinforce the stretching you do by sending those "good to go" messages to your brain. For that purpose, strengtheners that rely on body weight are perfectly effective. What's more, they are simple, don't require extra equipment, and fit right into your nine-minute-a-day routine. I encourage you to have a separate strength training program where you do use weights, but if that's not in your workout game plan, don't worry. The moves in this chapter have you covered.

A Word About Core Work

Many of the strengtheners in this chapter work the muscles of the core. Most people now recognize the word *core* as it pertains to fitness, but many of them have the mistaken idea that the core just refers to the six-pack of muscles in the abdominal area.

They think, too, that crunches are the magic bullet when it comes to getting a strong core. In truth, the core refers to the muscles deeper down that stabilize the spine and help produce force in the rest of the body.

When the core is weak, other muscles may compensate for the lack of strength and stability by stiffening up. And that includes the muscles in your arms and legs; if the middle of your body is strong, your limbs are less likely to be stiff. That's good reason to include one or more of the following strengtheners, which work both the superficial and deeper muscles of the core, in your daily routine. Each one will give you a lot of bang for your core-strengthening buck.

Working Strengtheners into Your Routine

If you are holding to the 4 + 1 formula I outlined on page 16, choose one of these strengtheners and add it to your daily stretching session. Even though I just stated my case for core strengthening, there is no right or wrong answer when it comes to which exercises you choose. I'll leave it up to you to assess your body and determine which area needs strengthening the most. I hope you vary your choices—maybe choose three different strengtheners and alternate days—or that you even go beyond the +1 guideline and add several of these strengtheners to your routine. Even if you are strength-training phobic, I think you will find the exercises are not difficult to do and offer great results.

Sets and Reps

Here are some common questions hanging over any advice about strength training: How many sets and reps do I need to do? What is the magic number? And how heavy should the weights I use be? All that will depend on your goal. Are you looking for more power, to build muscle, to ramp up endurance? These are the basic recommendations for each objective.

- Low reps (1–5) per set and lifting heavy weight = Power
- Medium reps (6–12) per set lifting moderate weight = Strength (hypertrophy, or muscle building)
- High reps (12+) per set lifting low weight = Muscle Endurance

Since most of the exercises that follow use only body weight, you don't have to worry too much about how heavy the weights you use are. When you do use dumbbells, just choose ones heavy enough to make the last few reps difficult. In terms of the number of sets and reps, a great place to start is with ten reps and one set, increasing the number of sets you do as you get stronger. Ten reps will give you an idea of where you are currently strength-wise, and then you can adjust according to your goals and the recommendations above.

The Core Strengtheners: My Essentials

DEADBUG

Granted, this abdominal strengthener's name doesn't evoke the most beautiful image, but you'll like how stable you'll feel when you do it regularly. While this is a dynamic move, there's no need to swing through it quickly. Going slowly through the motions will help you keep your back from arching and give you better results.

CUES

• Keep your abs tight as you extend your leg.
• Don't let your lower back arch.

TARGET AREA

• Deep inner-core muscles

HOW TO DO IT: Lie on your back with your arms extended toward the ceiling at shoulder height, knees raised and bent at a 90-degree angle. Tighten your abs, and press your lower back into the floor. Take a deep breath in. As you exhale, slowly extend one leg forward till it almost touches the floor as you bring the opposite arm overhead. Slowly return to the starting position. Do one set of ten reps on each side.

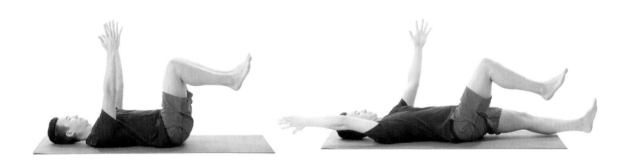

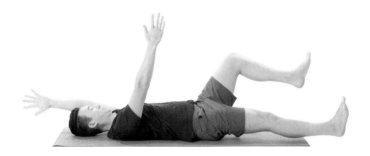

BIRD-DOG

Like the deadbug, the Bird-Dog calls for moving the opposing arm and leg at the same time. In this case, though, you do it on all fours, which brings in your hips, butt, and shoulders into the mix, while also allowing you to work your core. This is a very safe exercise, even safe enough to do when recovering from a back injury.

HOW TO DO IT: Get down on all fours, knees under your hips, wrists under your shoulders, back flat. Keeping your back and pelvis steady, take a deep breath in, then extend your right arm forward and left leg back as you exhale. Slowly return to the starting position. Do one set of ten reps on each side.

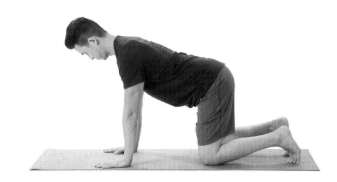

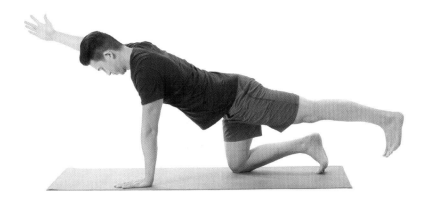

PLANK

Planks are comprehensive; they hit every abdominal muscle. The important thing to know about doing them is not to let your body sag. You accomplish this by tightening your abs and glutes as you hold, which will not only work your muscles most effectively but will also take some of the pressure off your shoulders and arms.

CUES

- Your body forms a straight line.
- Keep your abs and glutes tight to prevent sagging.
- Your shoulders are directly above your elbows.
- Your head is in line with your body.

TARGET AREAS

- All the abdominal muscles
- Glutes

HOW TO DO IT: Get down on your knees and lower your forearms to the floor, elbows positioned directly under your shoulders and your hands a few inches apart. (If someone looked at you from the side, your arms would form a 90-degree angle.) Step your feet back one at a time so you're balancing on your forearms and toes. Tighten your abs and glutes, and maintain a straight line from your heels through the top of your head, looking down at the floor. Hold for thirty seconds to two minutes.

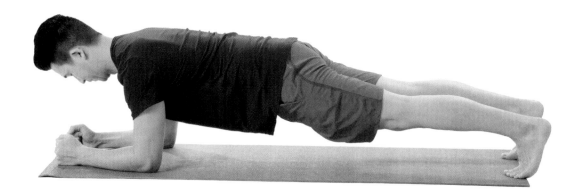

SIDE PLANK

This exercise provides the rare opportunity to strengthen the side of your body, a location often neglected by our usual forward- and backward-focused moves. Like the regular planks, side planks deliver when you avoid mid-body sag. Try to keep your hips from dropping.

CUES

- Push into your feet to help your hips rise higher.
- Your head is in line with your body.

TARGET AREAS

- Core
- Obliques
- Also hits shoulders and hips

HOW TO DO IT: Lie on one side with your bottom elbow on the ground directly beneath your shoulder and your forearm perpendicular to your body. Bend your bottom leg and place your top hand on your hip. Tighten your abs, glutes, and quads, then drive your hips up so your body forms a straight line from head to toe. Hold for thirty seconds to two minutes. Switch sides. Intermediate move: Keep your legs together instead of bending your bottom leg. Advanced move: Raise your top leg as you hold.

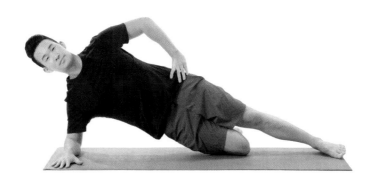

*

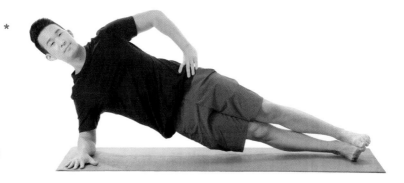

* INTERMEDIATE

GLUTE BRIDGE

The glutes are one of the most powerful muscle groups and play an important role in helping to stabilize the body. This is a great twofer exercise; the glute bridge strengthens the back of the body while giving you a great stretch in the front.

CUES

- Keep glutes tight throughout exercise.
- Keep weight on the heels.

TARGET AREAS

- Glutes
- Hamstrings

HOW TO DO IT: Lie on the floor faceup, knees bent, feet hip-width apart and flat on the floor. Place your arms by your side, palms down. Push down on your heels and hands, and lift your hips upward, raising your butt off the ground as high as possible; squeeze your glutes and pause, then slowly lower down. Do one set of ten reps. Advanced move: Straighten one leg as you raise your hips.

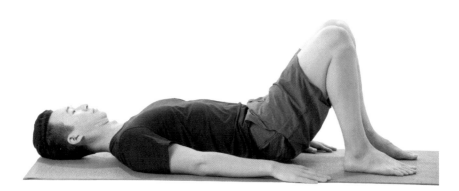

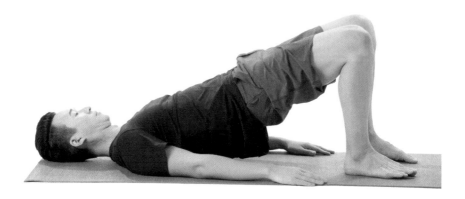

SQUAT

There is a reason you'll find people in gyms all over the country doing squats. They are simply the best way to hit multiple muscles, including those in the arms, back, butt, and (where you'll really feel it) the legs.

CUES

- Drop as low as you can go.
- Your upper body stays straight.

TARGET AREAS

- Quads
- Hips

HOW TO DO IT: Stand with your legs slightly more than hip-width apart (everyone is different, but this is a good starting point), toes pointed slightly out. Raise your arms in front of you at shoulder height. Bend your knees, and lower your butt as low as possible without straining your knees. Pause, and then slowly drive through your legs and return to the starting position. Do one set of ten reps. Advanced move: Hold a dumbbell vertically in front of your chest, keeping your elbows close to your sides as you lower down.

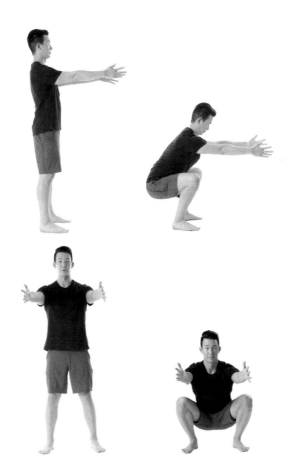

SINGLE-LEG SQUAT

Performing a single-leg version of the squat is a great way to make sure your legs are equally strong. Also, squatting on one leg allows you to work on balance and build stability.

CUE

- Your upper body stays straight.

TARGET AREAS

- Quads
- Hips

 HOW TO DO IT: Stand in front of a chair or bench on one leg with the other leg extended out in front of you. Slowly push your hips back and begin to bend the knee. Touch your bottom to the seat of the chair or bench and return to the starting position. Do one set of ten reps.

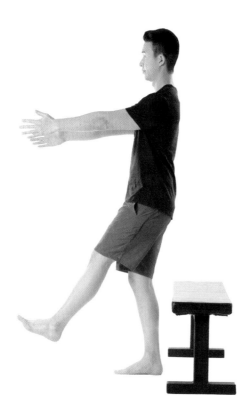
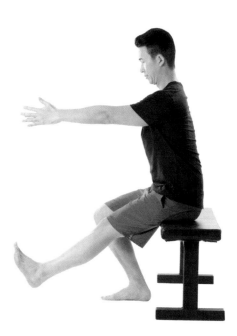

SPLIT SQUAT

The effort you make while doing this exercise is primarily concentrated in the front leg. However, being in that position also makes the body work a little harder to control balance and stability, so you really get much more benefit from the move than first meets the eye. Avoid bouncing when you do the squat.

 HOW TO DO IT: Stand straight, and place one leg a few feet behind the other, toes on the floor, heel up. Place your hands on your hips, and bend your back knee until it almost reaches the floor. Pause for a few seconds, then rise back up. Do one set of ten reps.

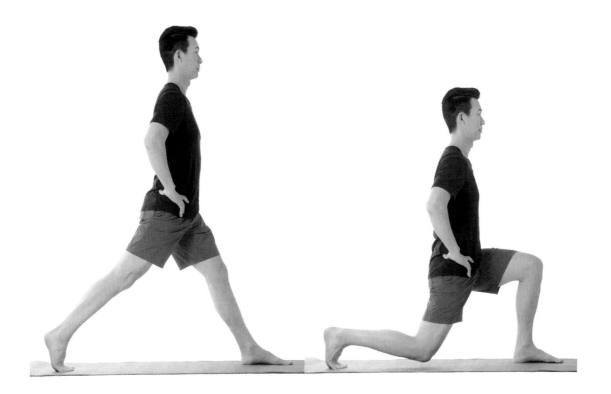

STIFF-LEGGED DEADLIFT

If the word *deadlift* conjures up images of giant-size Olympic powerlifters, consider that anyone can do it (and benefit from it); it's all about the amount of weight you're deadlifting. If you're a beginner, you can simply use a light stick. To advance, add in dumbbells in weight increments that align with your improving strength.

CUES

- Keep your arms close to your body.
- Your head stays in line with your back.
- Your movements stay controlled.

TARGET AREAS

- Hamstrings
- Glutes
- Back

HOW TO DO IT: Stand straight, feet hip-width apart, arms at your side, and a stick held between your hands, palms facing toward your body. Bend your knees slightly, then bend at the hips, and, keeping your back straight, lower the stick toward the ground just above your ankles. Slowly straighten back up. Do one set of ten reps. Advanced variation: Hold two dumbbells in your hands instead of a stick.

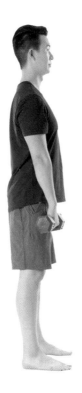

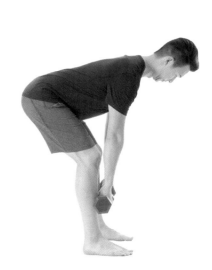

SINGLE-LEG DEADLIFT

While doing this exercise, you reach for an imaginary object—but it doesn't have to be pretend. If it helps, stack up a few books or pillows on the floor to give you something to aim for.

CUES

- Keep your back straight.
- Tighten your abs and glutes to bring you back up.
- Avoid opening at the hips.

TARGET AREAS

- Hamstrings
- Glutes

 HOW TO DO IT: Stand straight with your arms at your side, feet hip-width apart. Bend the knee of one leg slightly as you raise the other behind you, and bend at the hips as if to touch something (with both hands) about a foot off the ground. Slowly straighten back up. Do one set of ten reps.

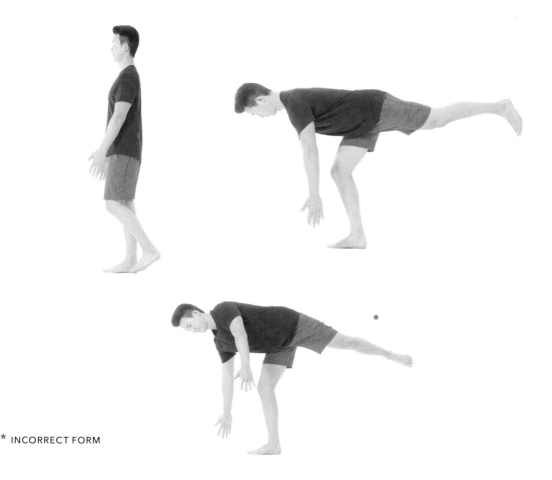

* INCORRECT FORM

PUSH-UP

Push-ups are probably the best overall upper-body exercise—but they can be difficult, so don't feel badly if it takes you a while to work up to doing any number of reps. And there are ways to make the movement easier, such as performing them with bent knees on the floor for support or doing them on a bench. Just know that, with practice, you will improve. And it's worth the effort, since push-ups do more than just strengthen the arms; they engage the core as well.

CUES

- Your body stays in a straight line.
- Widen your arms a little if it helps you raise back up.

TARGET AREAS

- Chest
- Shoulders
- Arms

HOW TO DO IT: Get down on your hands and knees, then slide forward until you are balanced on your hands and toes. Your arms should be shoulder-width apart and your fingers splayed. Bend your elbows at a 90-degree angle, and lower your body down to an inch or two above the floor, keeping your back flat. Tighten your abdominal muscles, and push up with your arms to return to the starting position. Do one set of ten reps.

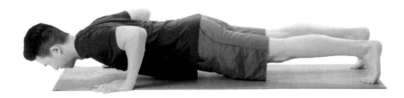

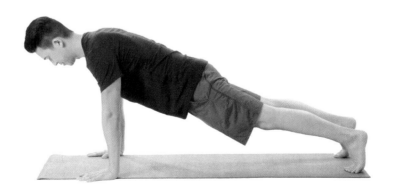

CHEST PRESS

There are many ways to do a chest press, but I like this one best because using dumbbells helps you work your chest and arm strength equally. As you get stronger, you can move to heavier dumbbells, or you can do one arm at a time.

- Holding weights with your palms facing each other is also okay.

TARGET AREAS

- Pecs
- Triceps

 HOW TO DO IT: Lie faceup on a bench. With a dumbbell grasped in each hand, palms facing up, bend your arms until your elbows are at shoulder height. Press the weights above your chest until your arms are straight and the weights are almost touching, then bend your elbows and slowly bring the weights back down. Do one set of ten reps.

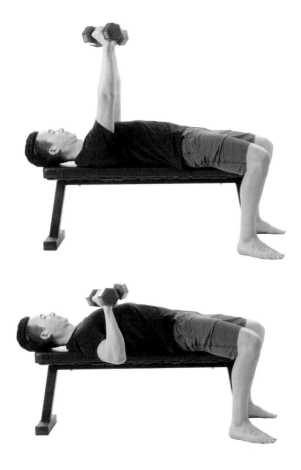

THREE-POINT ROW

The Three-Point Row is great for strengthening the back since, along with using your shoulder muscles, you also use your upper back muscles to "row." The payoff will be much greater than if you just use your biceps to raise and lower the weight.

CUES

- Legs are hip-width apart.
- Avoid arching your back.
- Keep your arms close to your sides.

TARGET AREAS

- Biceps
- Lats
- Upper back muscles

HOW TO DO IT: Bend over at the waist, back flat, arms reaching toward the floor, and a dumbbell grasped in one hand. Use your shoulder muscles to help you draw the weight up, bending your elbow until it's just about even with or slightly higher than your torso. Slowly lower the weight. Do one set of ten reps. Switch sides.

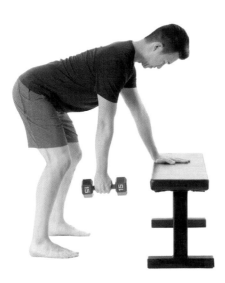
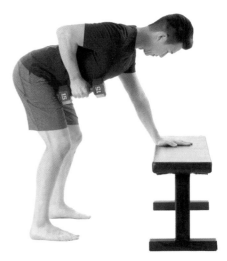

PULLOVERS

You expect to work your back and arms when you do Pullovers. Lesser known is that they also give you a great stretch in your lats as you pull your arms into the overhead position. The arc of this exercise makes it tempting to arch your back as you go. For best results, resist the urge.

CUE

- Avoid arching your back.

TARGET AREAS

- Shoulders
- Lats

 HOW TO DO IT: Lie faceup on a bench, arms raised at shoulder height with one end of a dumbbell grasped in both hands. Bring your arms back overhead, allowing your hands and the weight to drop lower than your head. Push up the weight to return to the raised position. Do one set of ten reps.

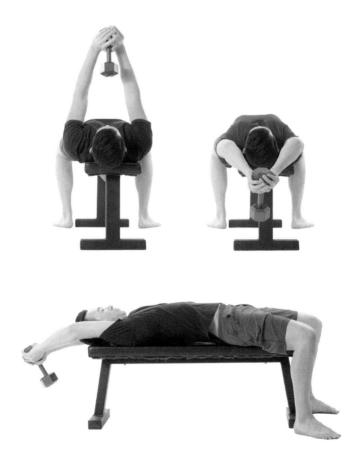

— 11

TOOLS TO ENHANCE YOUR STRETCHING

There are plenty of fitness gadgets on the market, but not many of them are reasonably priced and really deliver on their promises. Foam rollers—those cylinders that come in various sizes and textures—are a notable exception, so it's no wonder they have become as prevalent as yoga mats. They're everywhere.

I'm a fan of foam rollers and similar tools like therapy balls. I also love what I think is a great and comparable alternative: tennis balls. I think it's important, though, to be aware of what these tools can and cannot do. They can't, for instance, take the place of stretching. And I'm not just saying that because I'm the stretching guy! Exercises that use these self-massage tools are great supplements to stretching.

To my mind, foam rolling works best as a preworkout activity. Rolling muscles before you hit the gym or head out on your bike will increase their range of motion. You can do a little experiment to see how it works: Bend down to touch your toes and note how low you go. Then do some rolling on your hamstrings and try again. You will likely get lower than you did the first time around. The action of rolling your muscles increases circulation, which loosens muscles up. Follow up the rolling with some dynamic stretches—those increase circulation, too—and your body will be even better prepped for the physical challenges that lay ahead.

Foam rolling feels pretty good. Anytime you're sore from exercising or constant sitting or moving boxes or any of the million and one things we can do to end up tight and achy, rolling out the affected muscles can provide some temporary relief. Will it help you avoid post–physical activity soreness? That is a question still up in the air;

the research is inconclusive. But there's little risk in doing your own research. Roll your muscles after vigorous exercise and see how it works. Hopefully, you will feel less soreness than usual.

For all the good foam rollers can do, not all the benefits credited to them have held up. One claim that's been debunked is that foam rolling breaks down knots, scar tissue, and adhesions in the fascia, the fibrous tissue that encloses the muscles. Many people believe that foam rolling helps separate these bunched-up areas, but there's no evidence that such a benefit actually exists. What some experts believe happens instead: The action of rolling a tight muscle activates nerve receptors, which then send a message to the brain that it's okay for the muscle to chill out, at least in the short term. It's very likely that foam-rolled muscles limber up because the tool causes neurological changes that have a releasing effect, not because rollers break up adhesions.

Even if they might not change the physical structure of the muscles, foam rollers and other self-massage tools still offer a lot of value. They can increase range of motion, helping you sustain the gains you've made through stretching; soothe the discomfort of tight muscles; and provide temporary pain relief. That's reason enough to make them a part of your regular routine.

Tool Tips

There are tons of different foam rollers available. Some are smooth, some have grids or other patterns, some are wide, some are narrow, some are long, some are short, some have knobs, some even vibrate. The prices tend to range according to the complexity of the roller. The same goes for therapy balls. They, too, range in intricacy of design and price. I use a simple, smooth foam roller and a tennis ball for the exercises in this book and find they do the job well. If you prefer the psychedelic vibrating, trigger point–hitting ball and roller, that will work, too.

Which one you choose is a matter of personal preference and economics. There's no "best" one, but here are a few things to consider:

HOW FIRM SHOULD YOUR ROLLER OR BALL BE?

Everyone's body is different, and therefore everyone will have a different take on what level of firmness feels right (just as preferences for mattresses run the gamut). Your goal should be to find a level that gives you what I like to call that *hurt good* feeling—the kind of slight pain that feels good. When you use a foam roller or ball as shown in this chapter and it's too painful (hurt bad), that's a sign that you need to try softer equipment or change the way you're using it (see "How to Roll," opposite).

FOAM ROLLER VS. BALL

Balls provide more direct pressure on the area you're using them on because they're smaller. Foam rollers, because they have a bigger surface area, can hit more spots at once than balls. Assess your needs, then choose the right tool accordingly.

As you'll see in the exercises that lie ahead, rollers and balls can be used in all different kinds of ways. You can run them up and down a muscle, lie on them and go side to side, or simply press down to get some benefit. I'll show you how to maximize the effects by combining different techniques. For instance, a typical way to roll the calf muscles is to set your lower leg on top of the roller and move it forward and back several times. That will certainly help, but you can get even more out of rolling if you also roll the sides of the calf back and forth and if you pin the roller with the bottom of your calf, then point and flex your foot. There are many variations, and you will learn them here.

Rolling is a fairly safe endeavor; there's little chance of injury. But rolling should never hurt; if it does, back off.

There's no hard-and-fast rule about when and how often you should do foam-rolling exercises. If you can add it to your routine or use it as a workout warm-up, great. At the very least, do it whenever you feel tight or sore, and especially after any time you have spent hours hunched over a desk, driving in a car, or traveling on a plane.

How to Roll

Using a foam roller or ball might seem straightforward, and it pretty much is—but there is also more than one way to roll. The exercises that follow use one or more of these three techniques or variations on them:

Up and down: This is the most familiar method. You simply place the target muscle on the roller or ball and move up and down the muscle's length.

Across the muscle: Place the muscle on the roller or ball and roll side to side across the width of the muscle. To add pressure to the self-massage, you can also place one limb on top of the other.

Press and stretch: This combines two techniques. When you find a tender spot as you roll, press down on it and stretch the muscle. For instance, to press and stretch a spot on your quad (front of thigh) muscle, lie on your stomach with the roller or ball under your thigh, press down on the tender spot, then bend and extend your knee several times. Putting the muscle into motion adds a flexibility component to the stretch.

A fourth technique worth working into your rolling routine:

Press and hold: As you're rolling and you find a tender spot, stop and press down on it. There's no particular amount of time you should hold it; do what feels good.

Some of you may use a small roller, in which case, you will probably be able to roll only one leg at a time. In some cases, even if you have a large roller, I will instruct you to roll one leg at a time. Either way, it goes without saying that what you do on one side of the body you should then do on the other side. So, in every exercise, after you roll one leg, roll the other.

CALVES

UP AND DOWN: Sit on the floor with your legs extended in front of you, arms to your side, weight supported on your hands. Place a foam roller widthwise under both legs (or a single leg, if your roller is small) right above your heel (at your Achilles tendon). Slowly push yourself forward with your hands so your calves ease over the roller. Move back and forth several times.

ACROSS THE MUSCLE: Move the roller up to the middle of your calf or calves, press down, then roll your legs side to side to go across the fibers of the muscle.

PRESS AND STRETCH: Working one leg at a time, place the roller under the bottom of your calf, press down on it, then point and flex your foot several times.

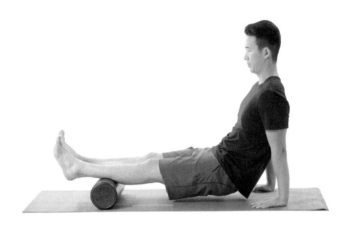

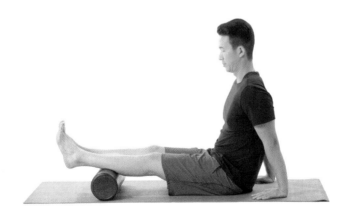

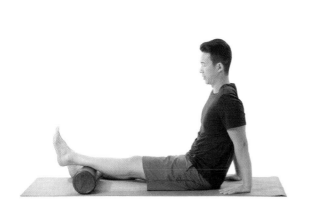

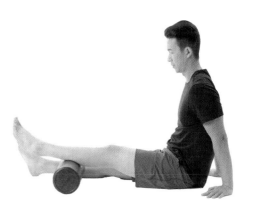

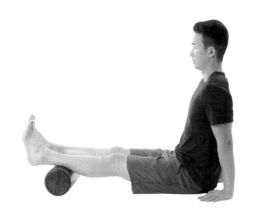

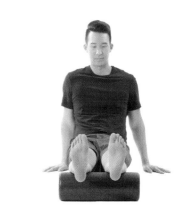

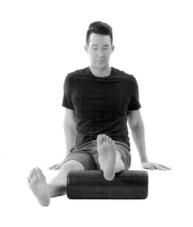

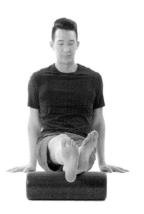

QUADS

UP AND DOWN: Lie on your stomach, upper body propped up on your elbows, and place a roller widthwise under the top of your thighs (or one thigh if you have a small roller). Slowly inch forward on your elbows to roll your quads, stopping as the roller hits your knee. Move back and forth several times.

PRESS AND STRETCH: Working one leg at a time, place the roller widthwise under the top of your thigh, then alternately bend your knee and extend your leg several times.

ACROSS THE MUSCLE: From the same position, with the roller at the top of your thigh, press down, then roll your legs side to side to go across the fibers of the muscle.

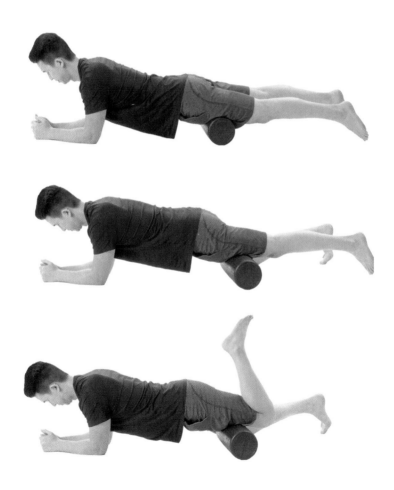

INNER THIGHS

UP AND DOWN: Lie on your side with your top leg bent at hip level, your upper body propped up on your elbows. Place a foam roller lengthwise under your thigh at the knee, then move back and forth on the roller from the knee to groin several times.

PRESS AND STRETCH: With the foam roller under the thigh just above the knee, press down, then bend and extend your leg several times.

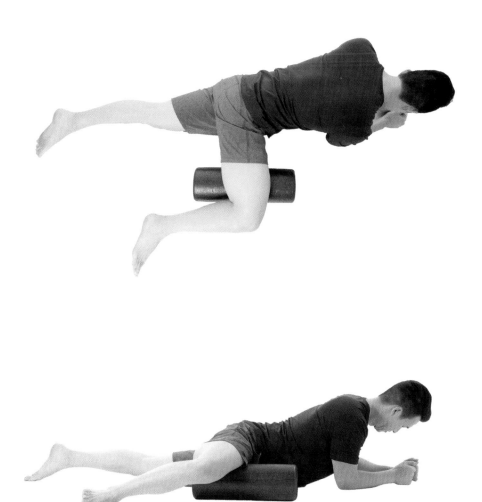

HAMSTRINGS

UP AND DOWN: Sit on the floor with your legs extended in front of you, arms to your side, weight supported on your hands. Prop yourself up, and place a foam roller widthwise under your hamstrings, just above your knees (or one knee, if your roller is small). Slowly push yourself forward with your hands so your hamstrings ease over the roller all the way up to your butt. Slowly move back and forth several times.

ACROSS THE MUSCLE: With the roller underneath the middle of your hamstrings, press down, then roll your legs side to side to go across the fibers of the muscle.

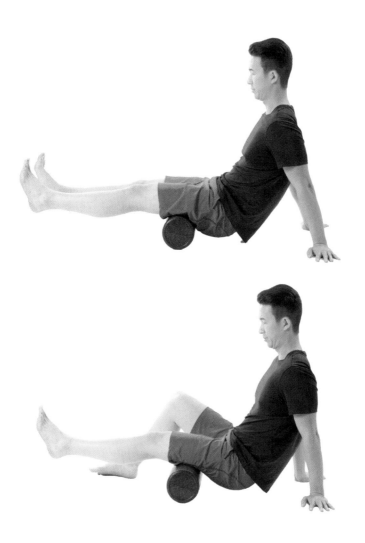

GLUTES AND HIPS

UP AND DOWN: Sit facing forward with one hip on top of a foam roller, the other hip raised slightly. Bend the leg opposite the hip on the roller, and place your foot flat on the floor. Rest the ankle of your other leg on the bent knee. Slowly move back and forth on the roller from the pelvis to the bottom of your butt several times.

SIDE ROLLING: Rotate forward slightly, and slowly move back and forth several times to roll the side of the glutes and hips.

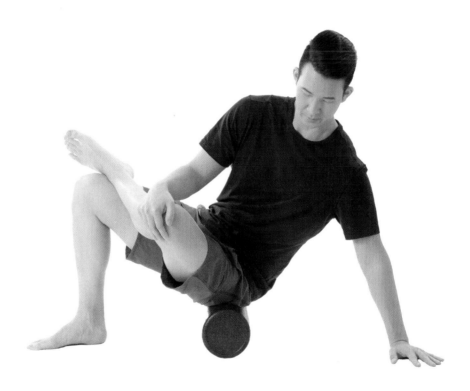

T-SPINE

PRESS AND STRETCH: Lie down on the floor faceup with your knees bent, and place a roller widthwise under the middle of your back. Clasp your hands behind your head, tuck your chin, engage your abdominal muscles, and arch your back. Hold for a good stretch.

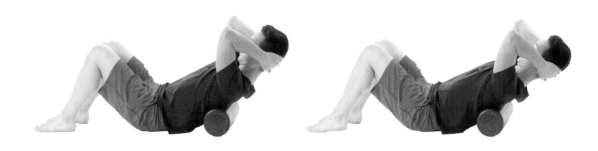

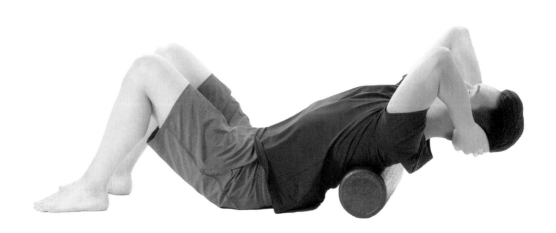

— 12 —

THE RIGHT ROUTINE FOR YOUR BODY

One size hardly ever fits all. This is as true about stretching as it is about everything else in life. Theoretically, we could all do the same five stretches and get something out of it, but why stick with a boilerplate routine when I may tend to get tight in a completely different area from where you get tight? And you may get tight in a completely different area from where your next-door neighbor gets tight, and on and on down the line. We are not exactly snowflakes, but our body types and our needs are fairly diverse.

There is also the fact that the stretch routine that's perfect for you on Monday might not help you accomplish the goals you have for Tuesday. If, for instance, you're feeling the end-of-week accumulation of tension on Friday, you may need a desk stretch routine, but on Saturday, the day you do your long run, a dynamic warm-up session is a better fit.

The seven stretching routines in this chapter give you the opportunity to choose the set of stretches that are both right for your body and right for your immediate goals. Most of them are made up of stretches from chapters 2–9, although I've added in a few new ones as well. The routines don't all follow the 4 + 1 strategy I outlined in chapter 1, but they each still come in at under ten minutes. You may find one regimen that you want to do every day. Great! But if you like, you can also mix it up by alternating routines from this chapter with routines that you create yourself from chapters 2–9 using the 4 + 1 formula. There is really no end to all the combinations you can stitch together. It will never get boring.

Seven Goal-Specific Routines

Desk Stretch Routine

For many people, there's no way around sitting for a good portion of the day. The kinks and tightness that go with being deskbound can be alleviated somewhat if you simply get up and walk around for a few minutes several times a day. This done-at-your-desk routine can also help immensely. It's very quick and doesn't involve any wild moves that will draw your coworkers' attention, but it hits all the spots—especially the neck and back—that tend to tighten up when you're perched in a chair for hours on end. Two of the exercises in particular, the Desk Cat/Cow Stretch and Back Arches, are designed to reverse the hunching that most of us do while working on a computer. I suggest copying these next pages and, if possible, pinning the copies up above your desk. That way, you'll be reminded to do them two to three times a day.

DESK CAT/COW STRETCH

HOW TO DO IT: Sit in your chair and scooch it back far enough from your desk that when you place your palms flat on the desk, the heels of your hands are close to the desk's edge. Sit up straight and tall, tuck your chin, then round your upper back. Hold for a few seconds, then reverse it; press your chest forward, raise your head, and let it fall back as you arch your upper back. Do ten reps.

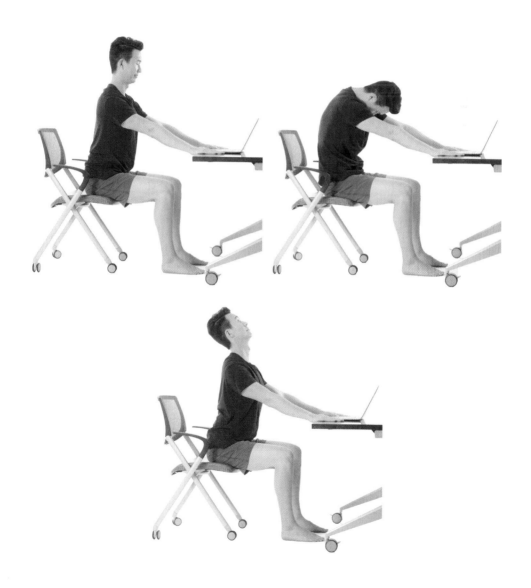

BACK ARCHES

HOW TO DO IT: While sitting in your chair, raise your arms above your head, palms facing each other. Scooch forward so your back is not touching the back of the chair, and sit up straight and tall. Arch your upper back, keeping your head and neck in line with your upper body (don't throw your head back); return to the starting position. Do ten reps.

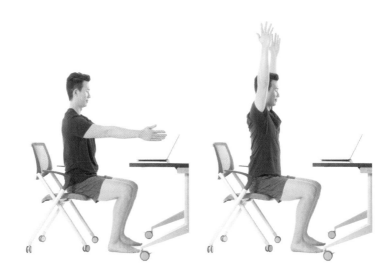

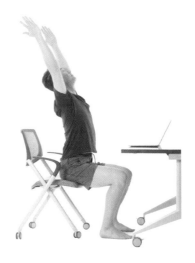

SIDE BEND REACHES

HOW TO DO IT: Sit up straight and tall in your chair. Cross one arm over your body, and grasp the side of the chair. Raise the other arm and bend to the opposite side. Hold for thirty seconds to two minutes. Switch sides.

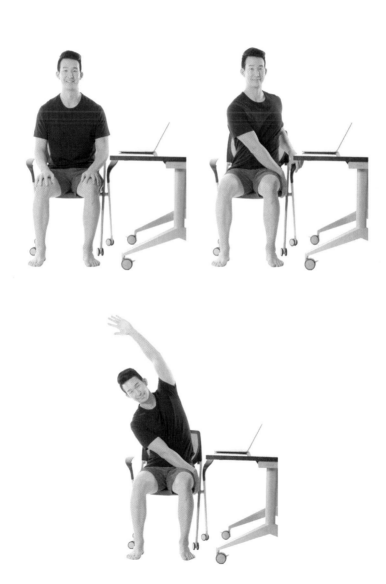

T-SPINE ROTATION

HOW TO DO IT: Sit on the edge of your chair and scooch it back far enough so you can place your elbows on the edge of your desk. Lean forward, and place your hands on your back behind your head, then push your chair back and sink your chest down. Lift one elbow and rotate your upper body to the same side, keeping your hands in place and the opposite elbow on the desk; switch sides. Do ten reps.

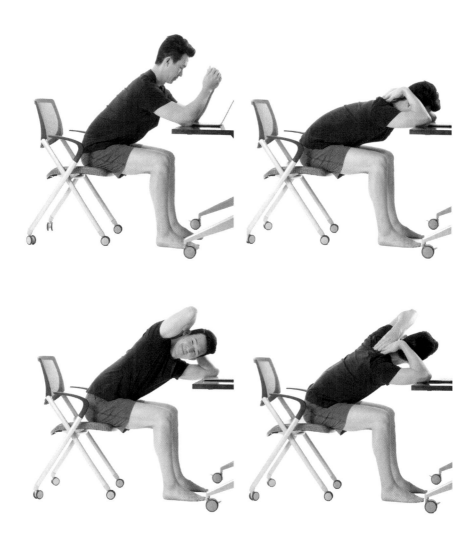

Dynamic Warm-Up

In chapter 1, I talked a little about the age-old question: Should you stretch before you exercise? The answer is yes, if you stretch dynamically—that is, rather than hold stretches, you move through them in a slightly more vigorous way. Dynamic stretching increases your body temperature, which makes your muscles more pliable and better prepared for what's to come when you begin your workout. The six exercises in this set are all combination moves. Go through them at an even, moderate pace, never stopping to hold any position for more than a few seconds.

WORLD'S GREATEST STRETCH

TOTAL-BODY WARM-UP

Stand straight and tall, then lunge forward with your left foot and place your right palm flat on the floor. In one continuous move, reach your left elbow toward the floor, then rotate your upper body and reach your left arm up toward the sky. Next, place both hands on the floor on opposite sides of your left (front) foot and straighten your leg. Switch sides. Do ten reps.

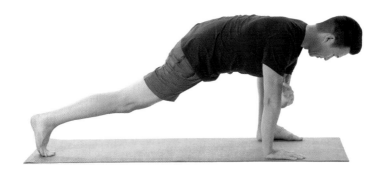

POSITION 1

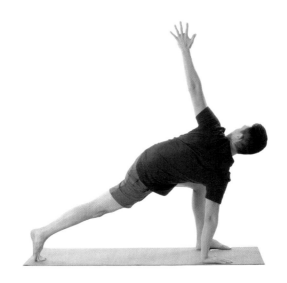

POSITION 2

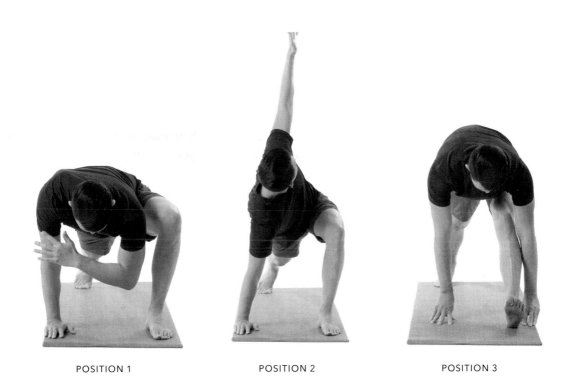

POSITION 1　　　　　POSITION 2　　　　　POSITION 3

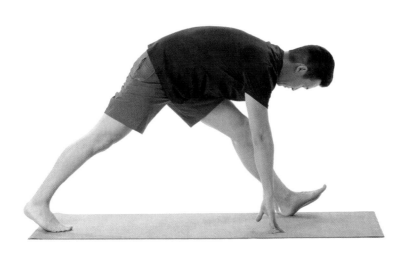

POSITION 3

WORLD'S SECOND-GREATEST STRETCH

TOTAL-BODY WARM-UP

Stand in a wide-leg position, bend down, place both hands on the floor, and walk them out until your body and arms are both straight. In one continuous move, push your hips up and reach your right hand toward your left foot, then come back to the start, bring your left foot forward, bend at the knee, rotate your torso, and reach your left hand up toward the sky. Come back to the start, and walk your hands back to standing wide-leg position. Switch sides. Do ten reps.

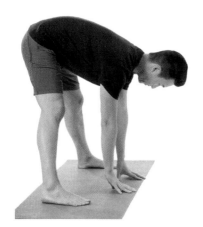

POSITION 1

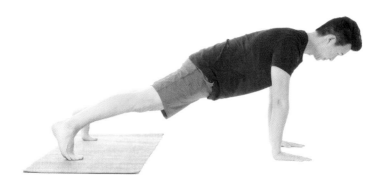

POSITION 2

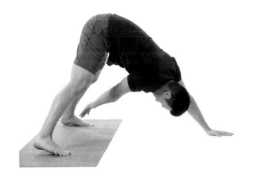

POSITION 3

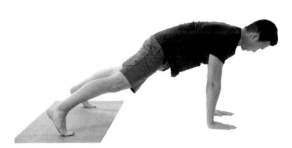

POSITION 4

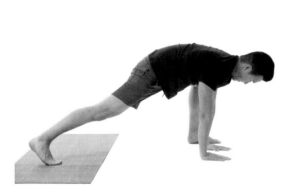

POSITION 5

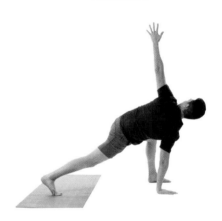

POSITION 6

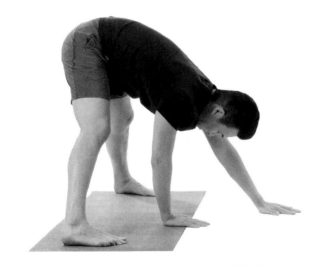

POSITION 7

KNEE-HUG TO AIRPLANE STRETCH

WARMS UP HIPS & HAMSTRINGS

Stand straight and tall, legs an inch or two apart. Hinge forward slightly at the hips, bend your knees into a quarter squat, and raise your left knee. Grasp the knee with both hands, and pull it toward your chest as you straighten your right leg. Keeping your right leg straight or with a mild bend in the knee, kick your left leg back, bring your arms out to the side, and lean your upper body forward in an airplane-like position. Switch sides. Do ten reps.

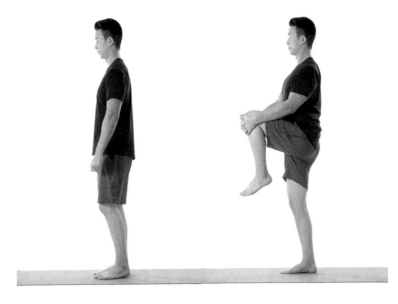

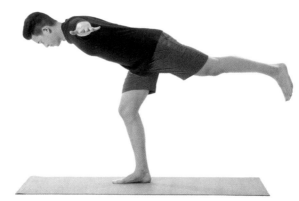

INCHWORM STRETCH

WARMS UP ARMS, SHOULDERS, AND HAMSTRINGS

Stand straight and tall, legs an inch or two apart. Bend over at the waist, place your hands on the floor, and walk them forward until your body is in a push-up position. From there, walk your feet forward to meet your hands—or walk your hands back to meet your feet—and return to the standing position. Do ten reps.

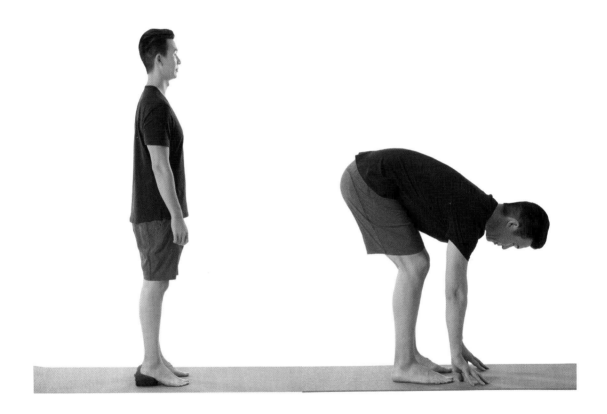

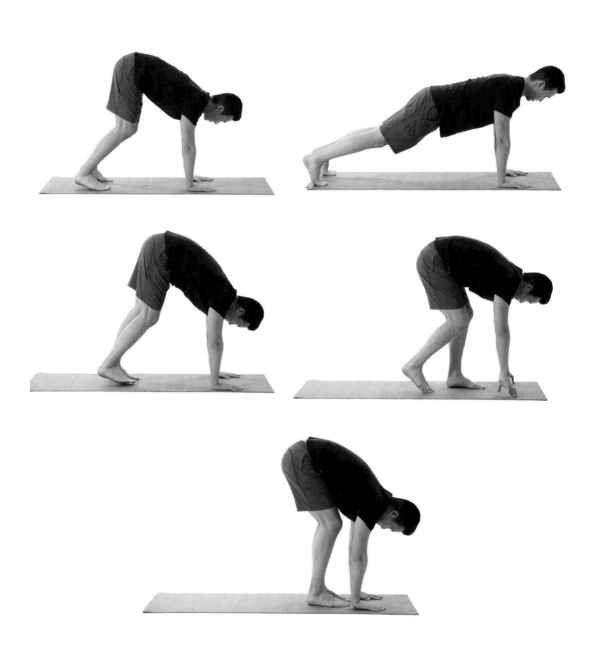

BETTER STRETCHING

FIGURE-FOUR TO SIDE LUNGE

WARMS UP HIPS, GLUTES, AND INNER THIGHS

Stand straight and tall, legs an inch or two apart. Hinge forward slightly at the hips, bend your knees into a quarter squat, then bend your right knee and pull your bent leg up toward your waist so your body creates a figure-four. Drop your right leg back down and out to the side, and move into a side lunge with your right knee bent and your left leg straight. Continue by standing back up and pulling your right knee into a figure-four again. Do ten reps. Switch sides.

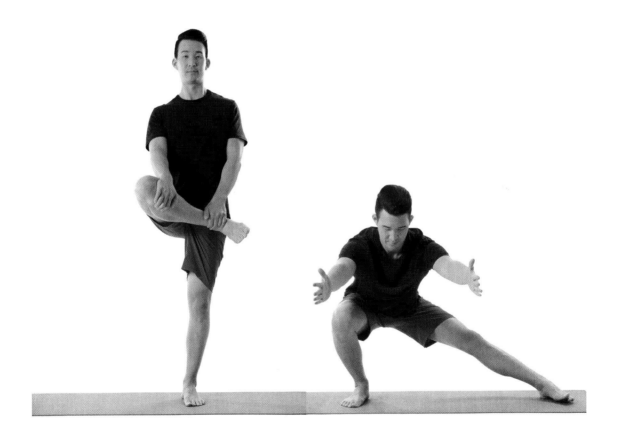

HIP FLEXOR TO HAMSTRING STRETCH

WARMS UP HIPS, CHEST, UPPER BACK, AND HAMSTRINGS

Kneel on one leg with the other leg forward and bent at the knee, foot flat on the floor. Slide your hips forward, and raise your arms above your head, arching your upper back as you go. Slide back, and bring your butt to your heel as you straighten your front leg and bend over it, fingertips touching the floor. Do ten reps.

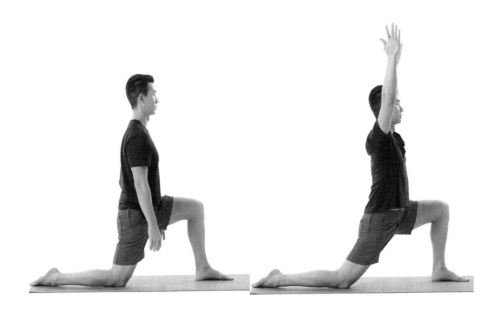

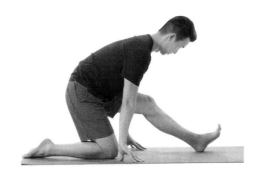

Post-Workout Cool Down

After exercise, especially if it's been strenuous, you owe yourself a little reward. I'm not talking about an ice-cream cone. I'm talking about some gentle moves that will help you slow down your breathing and bring your heart rate back to normal if you've been doing a cardio workout, or help elongate muscles that may feel knotty and overworked after an activity that primarily calls for strength. Mostly, a post-workout cool-down session simply feels really good, and that can add to the payoff you get from exercise.

- Any Figure-Four Stretch (pages 70, 71, 177)
- Hip Flexor Stretch (Half-Kneeling) (page 56)
- Standing Hamstring Stretch on a Bench (page 48)
- Side Bend Stretch (Standing) (page 98)

Low Back Routine

Most people will experience low back pain at some point in their lives. Not fun. Lower back problems can be a complex issue. There are many different causes, which is why it would be a reach to say that stretching is a can't-fail remedy for the pain. However, moving and stretching the muscles of the back and those adjacent to them can have a hugely positive impact on how you feel. These stretches for the lower back and hip area help take some pressure off the lower back so your movements are lighter and less constricted.

- Cat/Cow Stretch (page 82)
- Modified Hurdler Stretch with Side Bend (page 77)
- Hip Flexor Stretch (Half-Kneeling) (page 56)
- Pigeon Pose (page 65)

Looseners for Tight Shoulders

Tight shoulders can cause pain or stiffness in your neck, back, and upper body, and they may limit the things you do on a daily basis. The cause? It could be any number of things, but it mostly comes down to stress and anxiety (hunched shoulders are usually a sign these are in play), and overuse of some kind. This routine will help you target the area, loosening up the joints and helping to ease the tension.

- Pec Stretch on Wall (page 109)
- Protraction and Retraction Stretch (page 108)
- T-Spine Windmill Stretch (Half-Kneeling) (page 91)
- Wall Slide with Shoulder Lift-Off (page 112)

"Text" Neck Stretches

Look around and I bet that almost everyone you see has their neck bent, shoulders hunched, and head jutting out as they scan their computers or check their phones. This is such a common body position that the world is now filled with people who have cricks in their necks. If you are one of them, these exercises can help by elongating the muscles that surround the neck and reach down into the shoulders and back. And they really require no space, so you can do them anytime, anywhere.

- T-Spine Cat/Cow Stretch (page 83)
- Trap Stretch (page 127)
- SCM Stretch (page 129)
- Wall Angels (page 106)

Morning Wake-Ups

If you're like me, you probably feel stiffer than usual in the morning, and it can take some time for your body to get back to "normal." The best thing you can do to speed up the process is to move. The more you move, the faster your body is going to switch into its regular operating mode. What follows is a great routine for increasing circulation without shocking your body from its sleepy state. The stretches concentrate on getting the most important areas of the body moving so you can start the day on the right foot.

- Cat/Cow Stretch (page 82)
- 90/90 Moving Stretch (page 62)
- Hip Flexor to Hamstring Stretch (page 178)
- Pec Stretch on Wall (page 109)

Nighttime Soothers

If you tried the morning wake-up routine, you know it emphasizes moving to get the body revved up and ready for the day ahead. At night, though, you want to calm the body down and get it relaxed so it's easier to drift off to sleep. This set of stretches minimizes moving and concentrates on breathing into long, easy stretches. It will help you wind down, just what you want at the end of a long day.

- Butterfly Stretch (page 51)
- Figure-Four Laying Down Stretch (page 71)
- Child's Pose (page 75)
- Open Book (page 95)

— 13

WHAT'S NEXT?

Throughout this book, I've tried to drive home one simple message: If you've got nine minutes (and who doesn't have nine minutes?), you've got time to move your body in ways that are going to make it feel and perform so much better. Stretching can be quick and effective, so there's no excuse not to do it!

My goal has been to make it easy for you to establish a stretching routine, and maybe even add in some strengtheners and self-massage techniques as well. But if I'm being honest, I also had another goal in mind when I set out to write this book: Getting you to use stretching as a gateway to a more active life, or, if you're already active, as a tool for pushing your body to the next level.

Say, for instance, you're not an "exerciser." Maybe you just bought this book because your back is always stiff and your hamstrings crazy tight. Well, now that stretching is helping you feel better, why not ease into other types of movement to see if you can build on that good feeling? One of the reasons so many people start, then promptly stop a fitness regimen is that they jump in with both feet when they might do better to start by just dipping a toe in the water. When you take on too much—"I haven't run for years, but I'm going to enter that 10K next month!" "With my new gym membership, I'm going to hit the high-intensity interval training class every other day!"—it's easy to burn out.

Starting with something as nontaxing but effective as stretching is a good way to dip a toe into exercise. But once you've mastered it, what else can you do? What's next? I encourage you to explore what other physical activities will suit your style, and to approach them in ways that match up with your abilities. In other words, take it slow; Rome wasn't built in a day. Naturally, the more time and effort you put into any endeavor, the greater the payoff will be, but fitness is something you build up, one step at a time.

And what if you are already someone who works out regularly—or used to before having a setback? If you picked up this book to add to your exercise regimen, I am hoping that the stretches will inspire you to step up your game a bit. Stretching improves range of motion, which improves how efficiently you move. Ultimately, that will elevate your fitness level. Plus, working out the kinks and tightness in your body can help you realize that, yes, you can climb those hills you've been avoiding on your bike, play singles tennis instead of doubles, or add another mile to your daily run.

In the same way, if you have been sidelined because of an injury or strain, I hope that nine minutes of stretching a day will help empower you to push past what you thought (or have been told) are your limits. Many people are told that they should substantially restrict their activities, advice that makes them shut down and stop moving. While of course it's important to listen to your doctor, the more you move, the better you will feel and the more confidence you will have in what your body is capable of. Light stretching is a safe way to monitor your progress as you heal, and it gives you a foundation to build on. Let it put you on the path to working out at full capacity.

The great thing about the human body is that it has the ability to do so much. The great thing about stretching is that it gives you a little window into the world of possibilities. So don't stop there. Ask yourself, "What else can this body of mine do?" Then be prepared to amaze yourself!

— APPENDIX

THIRTY-DAY TOTAL-BODY JUMP-START ROUTINES

Some people like to make up their own exercise routines; some people wish they had a trainer to spell it out for them. If you're in the latter camp, now you do. The three plans here each give you a complete thirty-day stretching routine to follow. It's all worked out for you so you don't have to worry about which exercises to do and can instead focus on jump-starting your way into making stretching a regular habit.

Each routine follows the 4 + 1 formula I outlined on page 16; the main difference among them is difficulty level. You can start with the plan that suits your abilities best and even (unless you start at the advanced level) piggyback one routine on another as your skill increases. That means if you are a beginner and feel comfortable moving forward, you have three months of routines in your future. Of course, you can also stay with the beginner (or any) plan and repeat it again and again, maybe slotting in some new stretches or strengtheners—or one of the routines from chapter 12—here and there.

How the Routines Work

Every day of the week, you will do four stretches and one strengthener. It will take you about nine minutes, depending on how long you hold the stretches. (As always, the recommendation is thirty seconds to two minutes.) You should do them once a day, or even twice if you're up for it (twice is twice as good). As you read through, you will notice that each routine asks that you do the same stretches/strengtheners every day for a week. The next week, you'll change it up and do those exercises for a week, until the following week when you change it up again, and so on. The reason for that is consistency. Consistency is key to success in many things, including stretching. For one thing, repeating the same movements gives you benchmarks for improvement.

It's much easier to see and feel your progress when you're doing the same movements as opposed to a random mix of stretches every day. Repetition also gives you a chance to memorize the routine so you don't need to constantly refer to the book to see what comes next (handy if you do your stretches at the gym or while traveling). I think you'll find the repetition is helpful and, since you get to change it up after a week, not monotonous.

Where should you begin? If you are completely new to stretching, haven't stretched since your high school gym teacher made you, or don't do any formal exercise at all, go with the Beginner Routine. Try the Intermediate Routine if you already do some stretching or work out regularly. The Advanced Routine is best if you are an avid athlete. Whichever you choose, give yourself some wiggle room. If it's too easy, move up; if it's too hard, move back a level. As always, let your body be your guide.

Beginner Routine

This plan includes gentle stretches with an emphasis on passive stretching so the body becomes familiar with new ranges of motion. It becomes a bit more challenging each week as more movement is mixed in with the static stretching.

DAY 1–5

1. Child's Pose (page 75)
2. Hip Flexor Stretch (Half-Kneeling) (page 56)
3. Cross-Body Stretch (page 103)
4. Foot Stretch (Kneeling) (page 22)
5. Deadbug (page 138)

DAY 6–10

1. Cat/Cow Stretch (Seated) (page 85)
2. Lazy Groin Stretch (page 50)
3. Pec Stretch on Wall (page 109)
4. Calf Stretch (Standing) (Gastrocnemius) (page 31)
5. Bird-Dog (page 139)

DAY 11–15

1. T-Spine Rotation (On All Fours) (page 86)
2. Figure-Four Supported Stretch (page 70)
3. Finger/Hand Stretch (page 123)
4. Standing Hamstring Stretch on a Bench (page 48)
5. Plank (page 140)

DAY 16–20

1. Child's Pose with Side Bend (page 97)
2. Quad Stretch (Standing) (page 36)
3. Dynamic Pec Stretch (Half-Kneeling) (page 110)
4. Calf Stretch (On All Fours) (page 33)
5. Glute Bridge (page 142)

DAY 21–25

1. Figure-Four Lying-Down Stretch (page TK)
2. T-Spine Cat/Cow Stretch (page TK)
3. Wide-Legged Hamstring Stretch (page TK)
4. Biceps Stretch on Wall (page TK)
5. Side Plank (page TK)

DAY 26–30

1. 90/90 Moving Stretch with Support (page 63)
2. Side Bend Stretch (Standing) (page 98)
3. Hip Flexor Stretch on a Bench (page 67)
4. Trap Stretch (page 127)
5. Squat (page 143)

Intermediate Routine

This plan has more mobility stretches than the Beginner Routine, and it ups the degree of difficulty slightly.

DAY 1–5

1. Cat/Cow Stretch (page 82)
2. Hip Flexor Stretch (Half-Kneeling) (page 56)
3. Dynamic Pec Stretch (Half-Kneeling) (page 110)
4. 90/90 Moving Stretch with Support (page 63)
5. Deadbug (page 138)

DAY 6–10

1. Child's Pose (page 75)
2. Standing Hamstring Stretch on a Bench (page 48)
3. Ankle Mobility Exercise (Half-Kneeling) (page 27)
4. Levator Scapulae Stretch (page 128)
5. Bird-Dog (page 139)

DAY 11–15

1. Modified Lizard Pose (page 64)
2. Puppy Pose (page 90)
3. Modified Hurdler Stretch with Side Bend (page 77)
4. Forearm Stretch (Kneeling) (Flexors) (page 121)
5. Squat (page 143)

DAY 16–20

1. Groin Stretch (Half-Kneeling) (page 45)
2. T-Spine Cat/Cow Stretch (page 83)
3. Wall Angels (page 106)
4. Triceps Stretch (Standing) (page 118)
5. Glute Bridge (page 142)

DAY 21–25

1. Frog Pose (page 52)
2. T-Spine Rotation (On All Fours) (page 86)

3. Hamstring 90/90 Stretch (page 49)
4. Protraction and Retraction Stretch (page 108)
5. Push-Up (page 148)

DAY 26–30

1. T-Spine Windmill Stretch (Half-Kneeling) (page 91)
2. 90/90 Moving Stretch (page 62)
3. Dynamic Child's Pose (page 76)
4. Dynamic Pec Stretch (Half-Kneeling) (page 110)
5. Single-Leg Deadlift (page 147)

Advanced Routine

The next step on the continuum from the Intermediate Routine, this routine focuses on controlling movements to make them more difficult and thus more effective.

DAY 1–5

1. 90/90 Stretch for Hip External and Internal Rotation (page 59)
2. T-Spine Cat/Cow Stretch (page 83)
3. Hip Flexor Stretch on a Bench (page 67)
4. Wall Angels (page 106)
5. Side Plank (page 141)

DAY 6–10

1. Pigeon Pose (page 65)
2. Threading the Needle (page 101)
3. Groin Rocking Stretch (page 46)
4. Biceps Stretch (Kneeling) (page 115)
5. Single-Leg Deadlift (page 147)

DAY 11–15

1. The Brettzel (page 53)

2. T-Spine Extension on Bench (page 94)
3. Three-Way Hip Stretch (page 57)
4. Wall Slide with Shoulder Lift-Off (page 112)
5. Push-Up (page 148)

DAY 16–20

1. 90/90 Moving Stretch (page 62)
2. T-Spine Windmill Stretch (Half-Kneeling) (page 91)
3. Quad Stretch (Kneeling) (page 37)
4. Child's Pose with Triceps (page 119)
5. Split Squat (page 145)

DAY 21–25

1. Modified Lizard Pose (page 64)
2. T-Spine Extension on Wall (Tall-Kneeling) (page 89)
3. Hamstring 90/90 Stretch (page 49)
4. Scorpion Stretch (page 111)
5. Pullovers (page 151)

DAY 26–30

1. Tactical Frog (page 68)
2. The Brettzel 2.0 (page 69)
3. 90/90 Stretch with Side Bend (page 60)
4. Dynamic Pec Stretch (Half-Kneeling) (page 110)
5. Single-Leg Squat (page 144)

ACKNOWLEDGMENTS

I have to start by thanking my mom and my sister for always supporting me as I figured out what my purpose in life is. There were a lot of ups and downs involved in that endeavor, but you two never doubted my abilities, and this book couldn't have been possible without you. Thank you.

To my best friends, thank you for supporting me and always listening to what I had on my mind.

To my collaborator, Daryn Eller. As someone who spends most of my time in front of the camera explaining things, it's difficult for me to put those same words on paper. Thank you for taking on this project when it was only an idea and spending all those hours listening to me to find the perfect words to put in this book.

To my agent, Jeff Silberman, who guided me through the process of getting a book published. Thank you.

And finally, thank you to my editor, Elizabeth Beier, and the team at St. Martin's Publishing Group for making this book happen.

INDEX

3/20